PRAISE FOR

SILICONE ON TRIAL

"*Silicone on Trial* offers a meticulous and readable accounting of the breast implant fiasco, when an agency head's arrogant mismanagement wrecked an industry and needlessly terrified millions of women, behavior that reveals a pernicious form of government corruption."

— Henry Miller MD, Former Director, Office of Biotechnology, U.S. Food and Drug Administration

"A refreshing account based on fact and science, plus a vindication I welcome after forty-six years on the corporate side of silicone devices."

— Jan Varner, CEO, Specialty Surgical Products, Inc.

"A must read for surgeons frustrated by years of FDA paternalism, also for patients seeking truth about breast implants or any other silicone device."

— James Wells MD, Past President, American Society of Plastic Surgery

"A compendium of silicone regulatory horrors that reads like a Tuchman epic. When the author highlights government's inability to change its mind, observers of FDA misbehavior like me will nod in sad agreement. Silicone on Trial is important history for the science community, the public, and the media."

—Gilbert Ross MD, Medical Director, American Council on Science and Health.

OTHER HISTORIES BY
JACK C. FISHER

Lead Pencil Miner: The Rush for Yukon Gold

Stolen Glory: The McKinley Assassination

*Stopping the Road: The Campaign Against Another
Trans-Sierra Highway*

SILICONE

ON TRIAL

*Breast Implants and
the Politics of Risk*

Cover designed by: Siori Kitajima, SFAppWorks LLC www.sfappworks.com
Cover artwork by: Siori Kitajima, depicting a breast implant placed behind the breast gland and in front of pectoralis muscles.
Formatting by Siori Kitajima and Ovidiu Vlad, SFAppWorks LLC
eBook Formatted by Ovidiu Vlad
Cataloging-in-Publication data for this book is available from the Library of Congress

ISBN 10: 0986267929
ISBN 13: 978-0-9862679-2-5

Published by The Sager Group LLC
www.TheSagerGroup.Net
info@TheSagerGroup.Net

Patient Photography courtesy of Anne Wallace MD, Director, Moores Comprehensive Breast Health Center, UC-San Diego

SILICONE
ON TRIAL

*Breast Implants and
the Politics of Risk*

By Jack C. Fisher

THE SAGER GROUP

Artifex Te Adiuva

DEDICATED TO

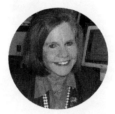

Elizabeth M. Whelan M.P.H., M.S., Sc.D.
Founder and Longstanding President,
American Council on Science and Health
1943–2014

"Spend ten minutes with Beth and you know
her integrity can't be bought."
WSJ, Sept. 19, 2014

In framing a government to be administered by men over men, first enable the government to control the governed; then oblige it to control itself."

— James Madison, The Federalist #51, 1788

"I think if this was exposed to the American people, say through a good investigative report, not only would it reveal some of the things that go on in Washington, but it might change some of the problems we have with approval of medical devices."

— C. Everett Koop, former U. S. Surgeon General, 1993

CONTENTS

11   Prologue

23   CHAPTER 1: A Bureau in Search of its Power

45   CHAPTER 2: Polymer Chains and Wartime Mobilization

53   CHAPTER 3: An FDA Validated and Empowered

65   CHAPTER 4: Silicone and a Patient's Self-Image

81   CHAPTER 5: Congressman Delaney and the Cancer Scare

95   CHAPTER 6: Regulating the Medical Device

107   CHAPTER 7: Balancing Clinical Risk with Clinical Benefit

121   CHAPTER 8: Dow Corning under Siege

139   CHAPTER 9: Silicone Disease? Or Silicone Victimization!

155   CHAPTER 10: Reporting the Rumor vs. Reporting the Evidence

165   CHAPTER 11: David Kessler and Naked Ambition

189   CHAPTER 12: A "Moratorium" and its Fallout

207   CHAPTER 13: Deliberating Science in the Courtroom

229   CHAPTER 14: Science, Regulation, and the Politics of Risk

245   Epilogue

255   Glossary of Acronyms

257   Chronology

263   Source Notes

313   Bibliography

327   Acknowledgments

PROLOGUE

On a slow news day, July 30, 1991, Minneapolis-St. Paul television stations received notice that U. S. marshals were preparing to seize a consignment of breast implants from a St. Paul warehouse.

A short time later, as reporters and television cameramen assembled in the parking lot of a storage facility leased to Bioplasty Inc, employees on duty inside could not imagine what had suddenly attracted such a crowd. There was no advance word of the action ordered by David Kessler, commissioner of the Food and Drug Administration (FDA). In due course, their curiosity was satisfied when federal officers arrived, flashed their badges, and presented authorization to remove fifty cartons of breast implants. Meanwhile, video cameras captured the action while reporters searched for anyone who could make sense of what was happening.[1]

The basis for this demonstration of government power was never fully explained by authorities. In a statement released to the press soon after the seizure, Dr. Kessler was terse: "Unsubstantiated claims mislead the public. They will not be tolerated." Several days later the agency revealed its objection to Bioplasty's claim that, because of an innovative translucent filler material, their "Misti Gold" implants facilitated x-ray examination of the breasts. Company officials were quick to remind the agency and anyone else who would listen that the device in question had been marketed since 1966 without adverse events. The required scientific evidence for their claims had previously appeared in a respected medical journal. Mammograms, they had shown, were more effectively interpreted when Bioplasty's product was selected over competing devices for breast enlargement. Because its device contained no silicone gel, it shouldn't have been grouped with devices recently embargoed by the agency.[2]

The FDA saw it differently. Soon after the seizure, an agency spokesman said, "This doesn't mean they [the implants] are bad; it doesn't even mean there is a problem. What it means is that they [Bioplasty] simply haven't filed a process with us." Indeed, the manufacturer had failed to complete the required steps for marketing an investigational product. Medical device manufacturers can disregard the FDA's bidding if they choose but only at their own peril. In this case no indictments followed the action, but the company was forced to endure the notoriety of widespread adverse publicity and eventually filed for bankruptcy protection. The regulatory issue in question had been procedural, not substantive; meanwhile, the enormous power of the FDA was again made apparent to every medical device manufacturer in America.[3]

Commissioner Kessler's focus on Bioplasty's mammary implant was a small facet of his broader concern for the safety of silicone gel breast implants. His evidence was limited to case reports of postoperative complications forwarded to the agency by consumer advocacy groups critical of any woman seeking breast enlargement. In addition, he was aware of corporate correspondence believed incriminating by attorneys already committed to filing tort actions against manufacturers of breast implants. The FDA's General and Plastic Surgery Devices Advisory Panel had recently examined claims of systemic illness following breast implantation and concluded that the evidence was very weak for some allegations and entirely lacking for others. The panel met in November 1991 and urged that clinical availability of breast implants be maintained while additional studies were conducted. Members of the panel understood that demand for implants came from women deformed by breast cancer surgery as well as from those seeking cosmetic enhancement.

Nonetheless, Commissioner Kessler elected to disregard his experts. Halting further sale of the products, he also called on surgeons to voluntarily refrain from any further implantation of the devices. In doing so, he elicited some of the most vicious attacks ever directed at his agency.[4]

By challenging the breast implant industry, Kessler ignited an emotionally charged issue, one that concerned not only thousands of women with their own private need but also several million recipients of other silicone devices. Because of the FDA's recognized authority, doubt was cast upon the safety of several hundred medical devices in use at the time. Spokesmen for more than a dozen medical professional organizations promptly declared their support for the safety of silicone devices, citing clinical evidence accumulated over the course of several decades. Many of them highlighted the biologic implausibility that of all the household and medical applications for silicone, only the polymer content of a breast implant should evoke a toxic reaction. Choosing to ignore these pleas, Kessler and his agency stood firm. "We know more about tires than we know about breast implants," he later announced. Meanwhile, his action energized the plaintiff's bar to seek punitive awards for many thousands of presumed silicone victims. Before court dockets were cleared of silicone actions nearly a decade later, more than $11 billion ($15 billion in today's dollars) would change hands, much of it passing from corporations to the pockets of attorneys participating in class-action lawsuits.[5]

The Minneapolis implant seizure was remarkably similar to an incident that took place in America nearly a century before. As dawn broke on a chilly October morning in 1909, US marshals waited in a Chattanooga, Tennessee, rail yard to intercept forty barrels and twenty kegs of Coca-Cola syrup due to arrive from Atlanta, Georgia. They had been dispatched by Harvey Washington Wiley, chief of the U. S. Department of Agriculture (USDA) Bureau of Chemistry, whose power to seize interstate shipments believed dangerous was granted by the Pure Food and Drugs Act of 1906. Wiley believed that the popular soft drink was injurious, especially to the youth of America. His putative toxin was caffeine, not cocaine that was by then routinely extracted from the coca leaf ingredient. Although the bureau's evidence for the beverage's addictive properties was inconclusive, Wiley and his staff based their action on newspaper accounts of Atlanta youngsters consuming soft drinks in large volumes. According to one reporter, "These kids all look a bit wild in the eye." Wiley had convinced himself that America's youth were being "doped on Coke." He maintained his position despite reminders that coffee, tea, and cocoa contained as much or more stimulant effect than was found in any soft drink.[6]

The 1906 legislation also permitted Wiley to use his police powers against willful misbranding of food products. He considered Coca-Cola's label misleading because the trademark name promised the extracts of both coca leaves and kola nuts. "Where," he asked, "was the 'coca' and the 'cola' in Coca-Cola?" Asa Candler, owner–proprietor of the Atlanta-based soft drink manufacturer, couldn't believe the government wanted him to provide cocaine to his customers, both young and old.

The enormity of power displayed in 1992 by Dr. Kessler could not have been imagined in 1909. Dr. Wiley's proposals to seize doubtful goods required the review of an oversight board, followed by approval from Department of Agriculture Secretary James Wilson, all under the 1906 law. Never before in America had a similar legal challenge been served on so large a corporation, one that was capable of spending whatever was needed to defend itself. The nation's chief chemist needed a victory to sustain his reputation, but federal attorneys knew they lacked evidence. Secretary Wilson reluctantly authorized legal action, and the landmark trial is recorded by legal historians as *United States vs. Forty Barrels and Twenty Kegs of Coca-Cola*. The verdict in favor of Coca-Cola both vindicated Candler's enterprise and contributed to Wiley's forced resignation.[7]

The Coca-Cola and breast implant seizures were orchestrated by qualified and determined individuals who perceived health risks they deemed worthy of action. Each was prepared to bypass the procedural inertia characteristic of their respective bureaucracies. Dr. Wiley was a prime example of America's commitment to nurturing its own professionals. He had taught college-level chemistry, had received his MD at Indiana Medical College, had earned a graduate degree at Harvard, and then had studied nutrition and food chemistry in Heidelberg and Berlin. Dr. Kessler is both a physician and an attorney. His prior government service was in the office of Utah Senator Orrin Hatch, and his administrative skills were honed while directing a medical center in New York City. Neither Wiley nor Kessler were lacking the qualifications or the experience required for their responsibilities. While some considered their actions to represent courageous leadership, others believed they failed to consider all of the evidence, electing instead to circumvent moderating forces in the nation's regulatory process.[8]

Throughout their respective careers, both Wiley and Kessler insisted they were entirely motivated by a concern for public safety. Each had chosen to move aggressively against business interests perceived to be in disregard of human safety at a time when supporting scientific evidence was incomplete. Not at all surprising was the resulting public outcry and subsequent charges that each had acted recklessly and irresponsibly out of political motive. Both incidents unleashed years of unproductive legal deliberation and called into question the efficiency of government regulators in a society that had traditionally placed higher value on commercial productivity than on personal safety.[9]

The litigation prompted by Dr. Wiley's assault on Coca-Cola bore no resemblance to the flood of legal actions following Dr. Kessler's campaign against breast implants. At the beginning of the century, passage of regulatory statutes yielded rules that were promptly challenged by the targeted industry. The Pure Food and Drugs Act endured repeated judicial challenges but gained power whenever the courts affirmed its legislative mandate. Decades later, attorneys wielded legal weaponry unimagined in Wiley's day. Although tort laws were enacted in the nineteenth century for adjudicating railroad workers' injuries, trial lawyers in the twentieth century learned to file suits against manufacturers on behalf of consumers claiming product injury. Announcement of a mere suspicion of risk from the FDA could lead to damage awards even in the absence of substantiating evidence. And whenever judges placed thousands of plaintiffs into a single group, called a class, a defendant manufacturer's only practical alternative to bankruptcy was financial settlement.

Standing In the background of both the Coca-Cola and the breast implant debacles was the problem of defining meaningful risk. If the basis for government regulation of a society's commercial sector is citizen protection, then how are risks to be measured and compared? Which risks among all the hazards experienced by mankind qualify for government limitation? Given the reality that some people are inherently risk adverse while others are remarkably tolerant of potential danger, then whose perception of risk should take precedence? The challenge then for public policy makers, regulators, and the judicial system is to find a balance between estimations of risk and restrictive statutory language, between product innovation and barriers to market approval, between unanticipated outcomes and reasonable punishment for avoidable hazards. Herein lies the basis for regulation being a political process rather than a scientific one, even when the product in question is based on technology.

My interest in these issues expanded in 1989 when I was asked to chair a committee of the Plastic Surgery Educational Foundation (PSEF) charged with examining for validity the many allegations of human toxicity resulting from exposure to silicone (polydimethylsiloxane), already one of the most widely used biomaterials for implantable medical devices. I had no specialized knowledge of polymer chemistry or biomaterial science beyond what every plastic and reconstructive surgeon learns during residency training and from subsequent clinical experience. My own research experience included laboratory and clinical studies of wound healing and the body's immune reaction to transplanted tissue. My expertise was thus relevant because (1) a patient's reaction to an implanted device is, like wound healing, dependent on inflammation, and (2) among the several alleged illnesses following breast implantation were disorders of the immune system. As chairman of the committee, I was asked to select additional members for their background in scientific fields related to the controversy. Fourteen agreed to serve, all of them with university appointments and proven records of research achievement. The committee also sought opinions from numerous consultants representing a wide assortment of scientific disciplines. Their professional affiliations ranged from academic institutions and public service agencies to independent and corporate laboratories.[10]

At that time, I knew little about our nation's regulatory policy traditions. After retiring from my primary academic career, I formalized my interest in the past with a period of graduate study in United States political and economic history. Readings in progressive era politics led me to examine more closely the basis for government oversight of commerce and more specifically regulation of the food, drug, and medical device industries. This historical interpretation of the silicone controversy caps that period of study.

Only from an awareness of historical precedent could I look back on a five-year interval beginning in 1989 and realize that I had been an active participant without benefit of understanding that the modern regulatory process is more political than scientific in its methods. I watched as the breast implant issue fulminated on television screens as well as in the print media, also in government hearing rooms, corporate boardrooms, courtrooms, and especially in consultation rooms throughout America where patients by the thousands sought relief from their worst fears.

The incipient event had come in October 1988 with a startling prediction of a cancer epidemic affecting thousands of women with breast implants. It came from Dr. Sidney Wolfe of the advocacy group Public Citizen, who knew how to play CNN for all it was worth, accusing all implant manufacturers but especially Dow Corning of withholding from the FDA their knowledge of this cancer risk. Omitted from Dr. Wolfe's prophecy was any mention of a decade-long clinical study, funded by Dow Corning and published two years before, that showed no increase in breast cancer among implanted women beyond the expected number.

Instead, Wolfe highlighted rodent experiments and demanded an immediate ban on use of breast implants.[11]

Reports of rheumatic diseases like scleroderma developing in women with breast implants prompted another wave of speculation and more panic calls from patients to their surgeons. Rheumatologists suddenly found their waiting rooms frequented by women with breast implants, many with arthritic complaints. In December 1991, when a San Francisco jury awarded $7 million to Mariann Hopkins for damages from a breast implant placed long after making a diagnosis of scleroderma, Commissioner Kessler chose legal evidence over scientific evidence and decided he must take action.[12]

Meanwhile, FDA hotlines were collecting reports of an expanding variety of symptoms developing after breast implantation. These ranged from migratory arthritic pains to unexplained memory loss, sudden loss of hair to mystifying skin rashes, localized muscular weakness to overwhelming fatigue, even leukemia and suicide. A mother in Florida facing charges of abusing her children blamed her breast implants for mental stress. Before the media and litigation frenzy had run its course, more than two hundred symptoms or syndromes would be attributed to silicone breast implants.

At FDA-sponsored hearings, bizarre scenes unfolded: alleged victims of breast implantation were often seen smoking in corridors, ignoring a proven risk in preference to an unsubstantiated one. Shortly after one woman was helped to the microphone to emphasize her disability, she was seen carrying her own luggage through the hotel lobby. One television reporter refused to speak with women reporting satisfaction after breast surgery, explaining that her editor had instructed her to put on camera only those willing to describe the horrors of their surgical experience. Women with complications were selectively featured on the afternoon talk shows. A *New York Times* reporter brushed off a spokesman for plastic surgery, declaring that a surgeon's self-interest was well known.[13]

Dr. Wolfe appeared at an FDA hearing in November 1991 to restate his prophecy: a silicone-mediated plague of cancer. Ignoring physicians and scientists poised to challenge his evidence, he stepped up to waiting television cameras where reporters offered him an opportunity to spread his warning to a national audience. At the time, Wolfe's organization was selling to plaintiff attorneys a $750 parcel of selected correspondence and medical journal reprints deemed adverse to the device industry. Public Citizen's objective was clear: to instigate as much legal action as possible against implant manufacturers.[14]

Initially reluctant to resist the FDA, professional organizations such as the American Medical Association skirted the breast implant issue but offered a statement in support of "clinically-indicated silicone devices." The American College of Surgeons and American Cancer Society, on the other hand, were unequivocal in their support of the silicone mammary implant for reconstruction following mastectomy. Meanwhile, the American Urological Association urged its members to avoid use of silicone gel testicle implants. Plastic surgeons, suddenly faced with a litigation crisis, had mostly forgotten that ten years before Dr. Kessler's 1992 moratorium call their trade organization had resisted a reclassification mandating prompt FDA review of the device. The petition failed and with it the opportunity for a thorough review of clinical experience long before people like Sydney Wolfe fanned the fires of controversy.[15]

Representatives of Dow Corning Corporation, when asked why they were not forthcoming with their animal research data, explained that their policy was to reveal what the law required, and then only to regulators. But the opportunity to influence regulatory policy and gain public approval had passed. Their concern for protecting market share might better have been directed at preserving the company itself. Plaintiff attorneys by the hundreds were poised to file complaints attributing several dozen adverse medical consequences to the breast implant. Further clinical study was made difficult because of incentives to claim illness following silicone exposure.[16]

The ubiquity of silicone exposure was well known to industry but not by the general public. In developed societies, silicone is inhaled, touched, and ingested by people every day of their lives. The food and beverage industries, especially brewers and vintners, rely on the antifoaming properties of liquid silicone. In any medical setting, patients receiving injections or infusions are likely to absorb microdoses because syringes and needles retain a fine coat of silicone. Any diabetic, administering insulin several times each day, might inject thousands of droplets over the course of years. Microscopic examination of tissue samples confirms a scattered distribution of silicone, independent of any implantable silicone device. In other words, the public's exposure to silicone had been cumulative since the mid-1940s.[17]

Yet the FDA's call for hearings on silicone was limited to breast implants, sidestepping the larger question of hazard generic to all uses of the polymer. Required by law to solicit testimony from a representative sampling of citizens, the FDA heard from recognized authorities as well a dubious array of individuals, many of whom were eventually shown to lack valid credentials. The agency heard from a few women claiming benefit but mostly from activists convinced that any woman with an implant was the victim of exploitation, either by a spouse or a surgeon or both. Naturally, the faux experts attracted the most attention from media representatives.

Judges presiding at trials involving breast implant manufacturers were not prepared to deal with the scientific questions raised. Few were capable of distinguishing between qualified and fraudulent experts. At one trial, elemental silicon and polymeric silicone were treated as if they were one and the same. A Texas judge declared the word "epidemiology" inadmissible: too many syllables. Juries were naturally confused by the conflicting testimony and issued verdicts based primarily on sympathy for the plaintiff. Compensatory and punitive awards in the millions were unprecedented and based primarily on illnesses defined by attorneys and unrecognized by medical science. Bankruptcies removed many device manufacturers from the marketplace, among them Dow Corning.

In the midst of this chaos, people were hurting, both physically and emotionally. Authentic complications of breast implantation were known to exist. Patients could be victims of inconsiderate surgeons who pushed the limits of tissue tolerance with exaggerated enlargement. Others learned their mastectomies had not been medically indicated in the first place, so it was easier to blame the implant manufacturer than to reverse the surgery. Most implanted women who developed breast cancer believed their devices were the cause. Arthritic symptoms are commonplace in adult women, but when they overlapped with breast implant exposure, panic ensued and legal action followed. Given enough of these coincidental events, class action litigation served as a powerful incentive for implant removals. Women without any medical issues sometimes became avid plaintiffs because of their fear of the unknown awaiting them.[18]

Now it became the FDA's responsibility to sort out the confusion it played a major role in creating. Nobody listened to the device manufacturers anymore; they were the villains. Professional organizations clamored to be heard, but the FDA wasn't answerable to them and believed that end users of implants only played a self-serving role. Meanwhile, Dr. Kessler remained in the driver's seat. Not even Congress could distract him. Tennessee Congresswoman Marilyn Lloyd, herself a victim of breast cancer, received no response when she asked why the FDA was restricting further implantation of a device the agency still believed safe enough to not require removal from existing patients?[19]

If Harvey Washington Wiley could have witnessed the enormous power wielded by modern-day regulators such as David Kessler, he might have puzzled over its remarkable expansion. This narrative begins in the final decades of the nineteenth century when Americans first asked government to rid the markets of impure foods and unproven drugs. The story of a fledgling bureau's attack on a major corporation is related in detail because a pattern was established for similar actions taken throughout the twentieth century, among them the assault on breast implants.

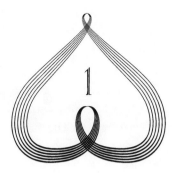

A BUREAU IN SEARCH
OF ITS POWER

"A government that tries to control what kind of food you eat and medicine you take will soon try to control how you think."
— Thomas Jefferson[20]

At the time of his well-publicized resignation from the Bureau of Chemistry in 1912, Harvey Washington Wiley was lauded as America's outstanding food purity crusader as well as reviled as custodian of "one of the worst Augean stables in any government department . . . where no scientific man can take the bureau seriously." Whenever the Bureau of Chemistry's achievements or follies were discussed, opinions of Wiley were anything but moderate in tone. Considered by his associates "a zealot for the public's welfare," Dr. Wiley always beamed approval for their choice of words. Meanwhile, he was ridiculed by the academy he vacated for government duty and remained controversial long after departing public service.[21]

Wiley was a product of America's rapidly expanding network of degree-granting universities and a prime example of the home-grown talent that late nineteenth-century progressives were summoning to Washington. The flaw in Wiley's character was an inviolate belief in his own version of the truth. Once his knowledge base in science was established, Wiley was disinclined to revise firmly held positions, even when faced with contradictory evidence. Because of swift advances in nutrition science and food chemistry, he was soon left far behind his professional contemporaries.[22]

Born an Indiana Hoosier in 1844, Wiley enjoyed a youth as rough-hewn as the log cabin he grew up in. His Irish ancestors had come to America in time to help vanquish the British at Yorktown, then moved westward to Indiana where they cleared 120 acres of forested land for cultivation. His parents were steadfast abolitionists who released their inherited slaves and hired immigrant laborers to work the family's land. The imperious manner that young Wiley displayed throughout his professional career was modeled after the authoritarian style of his Calvinist father, who supplemented the family's farm income by serving as both pastor for the local church and schoolmaster. Recognizing his son's exceptional capacity for learning, the elder Wiley first took Harvey to school at the age of four and directed him to remain all day within the limits of a chalk circle he drew on the floor. Young Wiley didn't just stay put; he absorbed every word spoken to him or written on the blackboard. He read history before he was seven and studied Greek soon after. His book knowledge grew at such a pace that in 1863, he was admitted to nearby Hanover College where he took an immediate liking to the study of chemistry.[23]

The family farm provided nearly all of the Wiley family's edible needs, and his mother's careful preservation of locally grown crops for winter storage was not overlooked by an observant son. Her aversion to canning with popular preservatives like alum and saltpeter required strict adherence to cleanliness, timely use of heat, and careful sealing of her jars. These habits served as one foundation on which her son would base a government career dedicated to enforcing America's first pure food law.[24]

Motivated by an older sister's decision to study medicine, he apprenticed for a year with a Kentucky physician before moving to Indianapolis. There he taught chemistry at Disciples of Christ College while studying medicine. After receiving his medical degree in 1871, Indiana Medical College invited Wiley to head its chemistry department. Flattered by the offer, he remained until Harvard accepted him for six months of postgraduate study, enough time in those days to earn a bachelor of science degree. While in Cambridge, Massachusetts, Wiley became distressed by a science faculty that supported the radical theories of Charles Darwin, all except biologist Louis Agassiz, who resisted the notion and provided timely comfort to the son of a rural preacher.[25]

Returning to Indianapolis, Wiley resumed his teaching but soon received an unexpected invitation to join the faculty of newly established Purdue University in Lafayette, Indiana. America's newest universities were adopting the German model for higher education, one that encouraged the integration of research with teaching, and Purdue's founders were recruiting faculty with that template in mind. Dr. Wiley considered himself well prepared for the challenge and became head of the Chemistry Department. At Purdue, he was considered a brilliant teacher whose independent research earned him the respect of science colleagues at comparable universities.

Throughout his nine years at Purdue, Wiley pursued his own research interests in nutrition and food chemistry. His particular focus was the processing of foods for mass consumption and the application of chemical processes to food storage. He became an authority on the varied sources of sugar, not only the cane and beet sugars, but also starch sugars mainly derived from corn. Granted a leave of absence, he visited Heidelberg and Berlin where he learned how a polariscope could detect variations in sugar content. His first scientific publication dealt with the food industry's habit of substituting less costly starch sugars (dextrose) for cane sugar (sucrose). Wiley disparaged this practice and dedicated himself to exposing corporate subterfuge.[26]

Industrialization in America meant longer working days for men as well as for a growing number of women. People who sat working at machines all day no longer had time to grow or cook food at home. Because prepared foods were often shipped from a distance and stored on market shelves, processors introduced chemical preservatives to diminish spoilage rates and protect profits. For centuries, meats were smoked to forestall protein decomposition, salt was added to inhibit bacterial proliferation, and pungent spices were used to cover up the foul taste of spoilage. The new discipline of applied chemistry offered many novel compounds capable of prolonging shelf life, not all of them yet tested for safety. Wiley's suspicion of the new preservatives and his bias against adulteration of food products shouldn't have surprised anyone who knew him. He didn't care what the intended purpose was—whether it be preservation, emulsification, or foam suppression—they were all wicked. He even questioned the value of adding newly discovered vitamins to foods.[27]

Along with his research and teaching responsibilities at Purdue, Wiley served as Indiana's state chemist. With his polariscope always at hand, he never missed an opportunity to test processed foods for their sugar content and declare adulterated any product containing starch-derived sugar. Wiley's unyielding stance earned him the disdain of corn sugar suppliers throughout the state and later the nation. Yet he never identified any health risk from dextrose. Meanwhile, he collected praise from a public largely unaware there were so many kinds of sugar. What people adored about their state chemist was his uncompromising advocacy for pure foods. Meanwhile, Wiley was learning that effective public relations earned him more praise than he could ever hope to receive from his academic colleagues. He cared little about criticism from other chemists. Because so many of them were consultants for the food industry, he assumed their opinions were based on self-interest and therefore invalid.[28]

Summoned one day by the Purdue Board of Trustees, he thought they might ask him to serve as the next president. Instead, they chided him for petty infractions: poor church attendance according to one member and conduct unbefitting a professor according to another—riding a nickel-plated bicycle through town while "dressed like a monkey." Wiley listened in silence, asked for a sheet of paper, then stunned the panel by scribbling his resignation and departing without issuing a single word in his own defense.[29]

What Wiley hadn't revealed to any of them was that his published studies of sugar "adulteration" had attracted the interest of Secretary of Agriculture George B. Loring. Soon after their meeting at a convention of agricultural chemists, Wiley was invited to serve as the Department of Agriculture's chief chemist, a position first conceived by President Lincoln in 1862. The offer thrilled him, for it represented an opportunity to expand his food purity mission on a national scale. At the time, there were no federal bureaus committed to health, therefore no means for granting or receiving funds for research. He left Purdue in 1883, proceeded to the nation's capital, and devoted the next twenty-nine years to government service.[30]

Dr. Wiley brought to Washington a spirit of reform as intense as any of the well-educated specialists recruited to newly established government agencies under Presidents McKinley, Roosevelt, Taft, and Wilson. It was a time of progressive optimism, when people hoped that the ills of an industrialized society could be healed with a political system led by knowledgeable men of integrity. Wiley brought with him his advanced training in chemistry and the food sciences, plus an academically productive experience in one of America's newest research universities. The personal baggage he brought along included several rigidly established ideas about food purity and an unrealistic agenda for what he might achieve in Washington. Disappointed to find that he was not the only expert in his field with strong convictions, the nation's chemist soon found himself at odds with scientists as well trained and experienced as he was. Furthermore, his critics were as committed to advising the major food producers as Wiley was to advising Congress. Business leaders prepared themselves for conflict with the government's expert by collecting evidence of their own.[31]

Wiley was shocked to find how meager was the Bureau of Chemistry's budget and staff; he had only five men to help him. Over the next seven years, he doubled their number and trained each one to function as both inspector in the field and technician in the Washington laboratory. Nonetheless, the bureau was soon overwhelmed by mounting evidence that dangerous foods existed throughout America's marketplaces. Even worse was the absence of any power to do anything about the problems encountered. Blatant examples of food fraud included baking powder contaminated with toxic levels of lead, "swill milk" from which the cream was skimmed and water added, and fermented wine diluted with water and sweetened with sugar. Food producers, large and small, readily admitted to use of untested preservatives such as formaldehyde, boric acid, copper sulfate, and benzoate of sodium. Spokesmen for the industry defended use of additives to prevent spoilage, citing other benefits such as improved textures, making processed foods more pleasing to the eye. Confronted with Wiley's resistance, food manufacturers demanded from him the science showing that their chemical additives were harmful to human health. Corn sugar producers asked the National Academy of Sciences to conduct an investigation, and its report listed no problem with the use of starch sugar. Incensed, Wiley declared the panel's conclusion the best that business could buy, a charge he made throughout his career. Yet he could offer no valid evidence in support of his own position.[32]

The Bureau of Chemistry failed to act on oleomargarine, or as a threatened dairy industry preferred to call it, "the greasy counterfeit." Entirely synthetic, the butter substitute was created as "beurre economique" by a French chemist, Hippolyte Mege-Mouries, who mixed skim milk and carbonate of soda with pepsin-digested beef suet, adding a dose of food coloring to mimic real butter. Wiley had little to say about the product when it arrived in America. Congress, confused about its responsibility, resorted to a time-honored practice: it placed a two-cent tax on every pound of oleomargarine. Protecting the public from suspected hazards with a restrictive tax became a tradition in America, the most visible example being tobacco, whose tax revenue is based on a product responsible for one of the twentieth century's largest death tolls.[33]

Without a well-written federal law supporting his efforts, Wiley could only dream of ways to police the worst offenders. His most powerful weapon was a pulpit from which he could embarrass the food processors and force voluntary reforms. He sought every opportunity to meet with reporters, issued his own press releases, and accepted every invitation to speak at public forums and to his favorite audience, members of Congress. Because he was personally fulfilled by praise more than anything else, he chose bachelorhood until later in life so that he might better focus on his primary mission.[34]

As a declared Republican, Wiley understood the need to survive changes of leadership that followed any election. He was first appointed during the Republican administration of President Chester Arthur and managed to retain his position when a Democrat, Grover Cleveland, took office in 1885. It seemed as if Wiley's position might never be challenged, until the 1896 election of William McKinley when he faced a new and uncommonly capable Secretary of Agriculture. James S. Wilson served in that capacity for the next sixteen years under four presidents, three Republican and one Democrat, a record for cabinet service never equaled since. Not a scientist by training, he knew how to listen and soon recognized the rigidity of Wiley's arguments. Seeking counsel from other sources, Wilson often reached conclusions contradictory to Wiley's position. Striving to balance practical and political considerations, Wilson displayed reasoning power that Wiley could not match. The outcome was a polarization that persisted for all of the remaining years they worked together.[35]

Legislation that might offer the bureau some clout was proposed in 1886 by Nebraska Senator Algernon Paddock. Wiley helped Paddock draft provisions that gave policing authority to his inspectors, including power to seize adulterated food products and dangerous patent medicines. Hopes were dashed when the Paddock Bill failed in the House of Representatives. Another two decades passed before momentum would build again for a pure food and drug law.

Throughout antiquity, food regulations were imposed either by custom or according to religious tradition. Civil laws governing food production date from the time of Hammurabi, whose codes regulated the growth of grains and determined wages for agricultural workers. Biblical dietary laws, as interpreted in The Torah, ensured public safety by restricting foods believed risky, such as pork and shellfish. Under Roman civil law, dilution of wine was a major offense. Pliny the Elder, who in modern times might have joined Wiley's food purity campaign, abhorred overuse of spices and accused apothecaries of spoiling nature's bounty with balsam. English common law demanded fair pricing for staple foods like bread, butter, cheese, wine, and ale. The Commonwealth Law of 1649 forbade cheese mongers from concealing rocks in their tubs of cheese.[36]

In 1850, Boston physician Lemuel Shattuck published a landmark treatise on public health and sanitation that cited alarming declines in average life span, from twenty-eight to twenty-one years! Shattuck urged the establishment of local boards of health whose efforts should "prevent the sale and use of unwholesome food, drink, or medicine." His findings attracted notice but failed to elicit action from Congress.[37]

Wiley's campaign against food adulteration was based on what might now be called zero tolerance for chemical additives of any kind. His effectiveness was entirely dependent on the pulpit he exploited so capably. But whenever he annoyed his boss, Secretary Wilson forbade him from speaking in public. Absent Wiley, the public could easily turn to the piercing voices of self-styled experts, among them Sallie Rorer, billed as America's "Queen of the Kitchen." Rorer's guidelines for proper nutrition made no sense whatsoever, yet she dominated the Chautauqua lecture circuit for many years.[38]

Ever since defeat of the Paddock Bill, Wiley realized that he needed better evidence that preservatives were harmful, not only to secure the trust of Secretary Wilson but also to capture legislative support for a federal pure food law. Returning in 1902 from a summer break in Europe, an idea came to him: apply the emerging methods of that day, prospective studies of individual subjects according to a defined schedule, later called clinical trials. Wiley's unique twist was to publically recruit experimental subjects, mostly government employees willing to place themselves at risk by consuming the alleged adulterants, since immortalized in the annals of government service as Wiley's "Poison Squad." Never convinced that the respect of university-based critics of the bureau could be restored, Wilson funded the studies anyway.[39]

Dr. Wiley soon fell out of step with the advancing scientific methods of his day. The new social science disciplines, among them psychology, were refining protocols for studying the responses of real people placed in experimental conditions. If Wiley was ever exposed to them, he failed to demonstrate any understanding as he designed the Poison Squad's madcap experience. What he did know how to do well was capture notice from the press. Fascinated by an exercise that placed volunteers at risk, editors assigned priority to the experiments. Reporters took note of the advertising for volunteers in which the purpose of the testing was revealed in advance. Alerted to the blossoming public relations campaign, Wilson summoned Wiley and made clear the testing would proceed quietly or not at all. The poison squad's valorous duty lasted five years.[40]

There might have been some truth to a few of Wiley's conclusions, but a lack of measurement cast doubt on all of it. Results appeared in Department of Agriculture publications, but none was ever accepted by learned journals. Wiley sacrificed his final chance to earn respect from the academic community. Yet he was admired by the public, and by enough congressmen to retain his post.[41]

All the while, Wiley remained hopeful for new legislative initiatives. He liked to think that his own research made some contribution, but the notoriety of his faulty experiments only served to impede a pure food law. Food industry lobbyists cited the absurdity of handing to a man like Wiley power to regulate their industry. Alfred Beveridge, junior senator from Wiley's state, offered to sponsor the Senate version of a meat inspection bill. Wiley sought Beveridge's support for a parallel food and drug bill, but the last thing the young legislator desired was to be upstaged by the popular chemist.[42]

In 1895, the first government controls were placed on packaged meats, in time to assure quality rations for troops fighting in the Spanish–American War. The bureau had declared safe small cans of meat despite an unappetizing gray color produced by chemical reaction with the metallic container. It meant nothing to Wiley, who was concerned only with adulteration. But soon after the conflict, the "embalmed beef scandal" made headlines everywhere in America. A day of reckoning would come when, in the presence of a sitting president who had eaten some of that embalmed beef, Wiley tried in vain to defend his blessing.[43]

Credit for passage of the Pure Food and Drugs Act is commonly assigned to Samuel Hopkins Adams for a series of articles written for *Colliers* that dealt with observed horrors in the drug industry. Honest labeling was abhorrent to the so-called patent druggists, inappropriately named because anyone applying for a patent would be required to divulge the formula. Hidden from consumers was the fact that most of these concoctions included hefty amounts of alcohol, cocaine or even morphine. Historians have long attributed enactment of the meat inspection law to Upton Sinclair's novel, *The Jungle,* a riveting exposé of the meat-packing industry. Sinclair spent weeks observing conditions in the stockyards of Chicago before writing a novel about the abuse of laborers in that industry. Released in February 1906, his book incited a near food panic; Senator Beveridge made certain a copy was forwarded to President Theodore Roosevelt.[44]

Now, with publication of Sinclair's book, everyone took notice, including the president who dispatched his Secret Service operatives to report back from the stockyards. TR sent an official

delegation to Chicago, and the Neil-Reynolds Commission reported conditions worse than Sinclair described. "Bully," exclaimed
Roosevelt when told of Senator Beveridge's meat inspection bill.
With the legislation now on a fast track, Indiana's junior senator
could at long last enjoy his coveted place in the limelight.[45]

Meanwhile, the companion food bill, sponsored by Idaho
Senator Weldon Heyburn, languished for months without progress. "The Senate does about as much in a week as a set of men in
business would do in a half hour," wrote one journalist. A political
cartoon titled "Bosses of the Senate," showed caricatures of key
senators seated at desks over which loomed giant cigar-smoking
figures labeled "Sugar Trust," "Standard Oil Trust," and "Copper
Trust." Bowing to pressure at last, Senate Majority Leader Nelson
Aldrich, himself an heir to a grocery fortune, informed Senator
Heyburn that he would withdraw his objections. Aldrich held
the power to swing all votes needed for passage in both houses.
On the day the Senate vote was taken, Dr. Wiley sat in the gallery
listening to 64 ayes and 4 nays. Days later, the House voted affir-
matively 241 to 17.[46]

The Pure Food and Drugs Act was the weaker of the two
laws signed on June 30, 1906. Regulation of meat was based on
premarket approval; every carcass had to be inspected before any
could be sold. Food and drug oversight was limited to informing
consumers so they might protect themselves from danger. A drug
could not be purged because of a dubious formula; neither could
a food product be seized because of a preservative. Only when
food was proved harmful or a label was found to be deceptive
could Wiley and his team act. Nor could inspectors proceed until
product was shipped across a state line. Worse still, penalties for
defective meat were substantial, whereas fines imposed on food
violators were insignificant.[47]

Roosevelt didn't much care for his chief chemist. Wiley's
impractical dictates brought long lines of annoyed visitors to the
president's door. And there was the embalmed beef matter. TR
was aghast when he learned Wiley thought saccharin was a poison. "When I told him this," the doctor later recalled, "President

Roosevelt turned to me, purple with rage, fists clenched, and hissed through his teeth that anybody who thinks saccharin is injurious to health is an idiot!" When the time came for Roosevelt to sign the food bill, Wiley asked for the pen but saw it handed to Senator Heyburn instead. Yet the senator's name was never associated with the law; for decades it was known as the "Wiley Law."[48]

Whatever passed between Roosevelt and Wilson, it never led to Wiley's termination. The president didn't dare fire him; both the public and the press believed the newly empowered bureau was led by a stalwart. Yet Secretary Wilson understood that restraints on Wiley were essential, so he appointed an oversight panel of experts, the Board of Food and Drug Inspection (BFDI), with power to amend the chief chemist's decisions. Wiley's reaction was volcanic, especially when he learned the panel included food scientists he had long quarreled with. "There was nothing in the food law authorizing this board," he fumed, and he was right.[49]

Wilson also insisted that legal approval must precede any interstate product seizures. When informed of Wiley's plan to intercept a shipment of Coca-Cola syrup, reports alleging cocaine lacked confirming evidence so the request was denied. When caffeine was later singled out as an adulterant, the BFDI asked why restrictions should not be placed on tea and coffee? Wiley never gave up trying, even risking loss of power he worked so hard for.[50]

Like Dr. Wiley, Asa Candler was born to a loving family and raised on a productive farm. Unlike Wiley, he was a product of the South and in particular the postwar South. The eighth of eleven children, Asa enjoyed the privileges of plantation bounty for the first decade of his life until war brought financial ruin to his father and devastation to Georgia. Unwilling to accept poverty as his destiny, he learned to trap mink in the hills near his home, strip their pelts, and sell them for a dollar apiece in nearby Atlanta. He also learned to buy straight pins and other notions cheap in the city and sell them for penny profits in the countryside. It was an important lesson; the beverage fortune he amassed was based on the principle that good money can be made on nickel sales to millions of patrons.[51]

Abandoning early aspirations for a college education and medical school, Candler apprenticed in a small town drugstore jointly operated by two physicians whose rural lifestyle and meager earnings convinced Asa he could do better in Atlanta, where as corporate legend records, he arrived in 1873 at the age of 21 with $1.75 in his pocket. Before nightfall on his first day, Candler had visited every drugstore in town, including the enormously successful operation of legendary patent medicine king John Pemberton. Finding only menial work with a competing druggist, George Howard, Candler reasoned the position offered him a chance to observe "Doc" Pemberton's enterprise located across the street. In 1877, Howard merged with Pemberton, and Candler became a salesman for Pemberton's enormously successful products.[52]

Meanwhile in Paris, a Corsican-born chemist named Angelo Mariani had popularized "Vin Mariani," a cocaine-laden wine beverage promoted with endorsements from prominent celebrities of the day: Sarah Bernhardt, Emile Zola, and Thomas Edison among others. Learning of the product's arrival in America, Pemberton essentially copied Mariani's formula and called his version "French Wine of Coca." Although an immediate success, the beverage faced impending temperance laws, so Pemberton removed the alcohol without relinquishing its buzz. Continuing to experiment with African kola nuts, he supplemented his syrup with its chemically extracted caffeine. Sensing that it packed too much wallop, he added water, lots of water, thereby enhancing the caramel flavor while also increasing his yield. With success imminent, he solicited a product name from his partners, and they came up with Coca-Cola. It was euphonious, and it flagged the beverage's two primary ingredients.

Pemberton thought everybody, children and adults included, should enjoy his beverage whenever they needed a "pick up" or a "refreshing pause," phrases that would annotate product marketing for decades to come. Envisioning nothing less than the greatest beverage market ever conceived in America or anywhere

else, Pemberton was quickly proved correct. Candler, in the meantime, was smart enough to marry his boss's daughter, assume
possession of his own drugstore, and soon after purchase a controlling interest in Pemberton's beverage.[53]

The appropriate descriptor for growth of Candler's Coca-
Cola Company is meteoric; few commercial enterprises in history
have taken off as fast as his did and then keep growing and growing. But despite partners who provided him with an efficient
operation for the remainder of his business career, Candler faced
continuing scrutiny from government regulators, among them
Wiley. Residual cocaine in the coca nut extract required a method
for removal conceived by chemists at the Schaefer Alkaloid Works
in Maywood, New Jersey. Because Candler insisted on claiming a
medicinal benefit, taxes were imposed that he later challenged in
court. After a jury ruled the amount of caffeine in Coke insufficient to be classed as a drug, he reaped a nice tax refund, but his
beverage remained within Wiley's jurisdiction.[54]

Executives at Coca-Cola kept watch of the pure food bill as
it advanced through the legislative process. Like most of the large
beverage producers, Candler supported the prospective law's provisions. Privately, however, he didn't relish having to deal with
any government agency, especially one led by a Yankee. Based on
prior interaction with the bureau, Candler assumed he would be
haggling over the chemical residuals in his concentrate, yet he
sincerely believed he had taken all necessary initiatives to protect
the health of his consumers. Because nobody could possibly know
his business as well as he did, how could any law dictate the way
he should conduct his enterprise?[55]

Despite Secretary Wilson's warning to leave Coca-Cola alone,
Wiley dispatched his inspectors to the Atlanta production facilities
time and again. Learning how vigorous Candler's protestations
were, Wiley sent his inspectors even more often and without notification. In July 1909, one of Wiley's inspectors returned with a
sample of the secret concentrate for laboratory analysis. Three
months later, Candler was informed that government agents had
seized a shipment of syrup as it arrived in Chattanooga. The feisty

beverage mogul immediately set to preparing for the most challenging legal battle of his career.

Learning that federal attorneys intended to plead for misbranding—in other words, failing to deliver the "promised" derivatives of coca nuts—Candler couldn't believe Wiley was punishing him for not putting addictive codeine in Coca-Cola. He had paid a high price to remove the drug from his secret formula. Although it would have been easy to do so, no record exists of Coca-Cola subverting the government's case by offering to reduce the amount of caffeine in each glass of Coke. Compromise was not an operative word in either man's vocabulary.[56]

For the first time, Wiley and his as yet impotent bureau had taken on a corporation large enough to spend whatever it took to win. The action wasn't made any easier when Secretary Wilson insisted the trial be conducted in Chattanooga where the problematic syrup lay sweltering in a warehouse. Wiley pleaded in vain that a trial in any Southern city was akin to fighting Asa Candler in his own back yard and risking a loss.[57]

Department of Justice attorneys preparing for trial didn't think they could be ready for several months. Disinclined to trust Wiley as their prime witness, they recruited experts from other government laboratories. Coca-Cola's defense attorneys took advantage of the delay by recruiting an equally impressive cast of witnesses, most of them from distinguished academic institutions. Candler believed the delay offered him time to gather better evidence. He instructed his lawyers to find a respected scientist to conduct studies that might strengthen the company's position in court. Candler wanted someone who could testify in a courtroom that he had actually studied the effects of caffeine on human brain function and then explain his findings so a jury could understand them. Coca-Cola attorneys found Professor James McKeen Cattell, a distinguished psychologist at Columbia University, who offered one of his best students, Harry Hollingworth, a talented young psychologist and instructor at Barnard College.[58]

Hollingworth had completed his doctorate in psychology under Cattell two years before. Recently married to a fellow graduate student, their combined annual income was little more than one thousand dollars, barely enough to get by in New York City. An honorarium from Coca-Cola would instantly resolve their financial predicament, but Hollingworth was wary of the assignment and its possible impact on his career. Yet he was equally fascinated by the problem; nothing quite like it had been tackled before. Negotiating with Candler's attorneys, the scientist stipulated that his findings be published regardless of the outcome. Furthermore, if the results were favorable to Coca-Cola, neither his name nor his university could be used for advertising. Candler and Coca-Cola agreed without objection.[59]

The contract proved a windfall for both Hollingworths. His wife conducted many of the studies during a temporary break from her own schooling. The sum paid to Hollingworth was never revealed by the parties involved, but in correspondence with her family back in Nebraska, she reported, "We did a big experiment for the Coca-Cola Company and made a neat wad of money."[60]

Hollingworth knew that prior studies of caffeine's effects were limited to measuring basic motor responses; he wanted to examine caffeine's influence on mental functioning. Sixteen graduate students were recruited as subjects, all of whom agreed to abstain from caffeine or alcohol for the study's duration. One-half swallowed measured doses of caffeine in capsule form, while the rest consumed a placebo capsule filled with milk powder and sugar. Allowing time for absorption and maximum pharmacologic effect, tests were conducted for perception, association, attention span, judgment, discrimination, and reaction time. All subjects recorded their level of daytime wakefulness and the duration of their overnight sleep. At completion, there were sixty-four thousand recorded test reactions.[61]

Just like studies involving the poison squad, each subject served as his own control. Unlike Wiley's protocol, Hollingworth's study was double-blinded, meaning that neither the subject nor those conducting the experiments knew what their capsules contained. This effectively separated the two principal investigators from any foreknowledge of the experiment's most important variable. As opening arguments were heard in a Chattanooga courtroom, the Hollingworths were still interpreting their data in New York. Neither Candler nor his attorneys were yet aware of the experiment's outcome.[62]

The Coca-Cola trial represented as grand a media event as could be produced in a Southern city in 1911. Reporters from Atlanta's several newspapers fought their local colleagues for seats in the gallery. Newspapers each day devoted their front pages to a full accounting of the prior day's testimony, with emphasis placed on the cross-examination and any comments from the judge. Most days, the courtroom was filled beyond capacity with local citizens desiring entertainment, politicians from as far as Atlanta, and attorneys anxious to hear legal arguments beyond their scope of practice. Unlike today, expert witnesses could listen to all testimony offered in advance of their own.[63]

According to the government's prosecutors, the case against Coca-Cola was based on five points. First, the beverage was adulterated by virtue of it containing an added ingredient—caffeine—a well-known deleterious substance. Second, the product was misbranded by virtue of its label promising a quantity of coca leaf derivatives not present following laboratory analysis. Third, the same argument for misbranding was applied to the absence of kola nuts. Fourth, the product was caramel colored, a deliberate effort to deceive the buyer. Fifth, the use of pictures of coca leaves on the label also served as a promise of content unfulfilled. Federal attorneys assured the jury they would offer ample evidence of the dangers of caffeine, including animal experiments demonstrating the substance's lethal potential.[64]

J. B. Sizer then stood and outlined Coca-Cola's defense founded on proving the United States government held no valid jurisdiction in the matter because there had been no adulteration and no misbranding. Therefore, the property must be returned along with accumulated penalties due, plus full payment of defense and court costs. Responding to the charge of adulteration, Sizer would first prove that caffeine was not deleterious in the quantities consumed by the consumers of Coca-Cola. Second, that it could not be an adulterant because it was an integral component of the original formula. With respect to the alleged misbranding, the name Coca-Cola had been trademarked since 1892 and was well known to all Americans. Any charge of deception was therefore ridiculous. Judge Sanford spent the afternoon pounding his gavel to reestablish order among spectators who mostly reacted as if they were attending a circus.

Despite the time and care devoted to their selection, the government's experts fared badly, especially under the withering cross-examination of Sizer. For example, Dr. Henry Rusby, professor of materia medica at New York College of Pharmacy and a longstanding consultant to Wiley's Bureau of Chemistry, admitted under cross that his experimental rabbits had been fed nothing but concentrated Coca-Cola syrup. Asked what might be the outcome of feeding humans nothing but undiluted Coca-Cola syrup, the question brought howls of laughter from the gallery and more rapping of the judge's gavel. When Coca-Cola's turn came, Sizer wasted no time on testimonials and called Dr. Hollingworth to the stand. The doctor's soft voice brought immediate stillness to the room so his every word could be heard. He methodically outlined the design and conduct of his experiment, explained what a controlled experiment meant, and emphasizing the measures taken to eliminate bias. This was all information foreign to courtrooms of that day. Had Dr. Wiley chosen to be present, he might have learned something about emerging standards for clinical research.

Dr. Hollingworth was not interrupted by either legal team that morning. Enumerating each of his test findings, he summarized that caffeine was nothing more than a mild stimulant whose influence on mental alertness was gradual but short-lived. His final conclusion was that caffeine, in quantities found in soft drinks such as Coca-Cola, showed no deleterious effects on mental performance. There was no cross-examination of Hollingworth; federal attorneys wanted him off the stand as soon as possible. Questions about the witness's financial link with Coca-Cola were never asked, and no one present ever learned that the ink was barely dry on the doctor's summary data.[65]

Believing the defense was in a strong position, Sizer planned to move for a directed verdict, meaning the judge would instruct the jury to return a defense verdict based on a lack of prosecutorial evidence. Meanwhile, federal attorneys didn't want their unconvincing case to go to a Chattanooga jury; they stood a better chance of success before three appellate judges. Learning the next morning that Coca-Cola wanted a directed verdict, they concealed their pleasure and awaited the judge's opinion. Sanford approved the defense petition on the counts of adulteration and misbranding. There was no adulteration, he declared, because caffeine was a natural component of the original formula. And there was no misbranding because Coca-Cola was a distinctive and well-known name. He took no position on caffeine's physical effect on the beverage's consumers.[66]

The Sixth Circuit Court of Appeals in Cincinnati, Ohio, later delivered a verdict upholding Judge Sanford's decision. Although Candler had been ecstatic following his "victory" in Chattanooga, his attorneys cautioned him not to issue statements because the caffeine issue had not yet been addressed. After the appellate confirmation however, there was no holding him back. Candler ordered pamphlets with titles like *Truth, Justice, and Coca-Cola*. His intent was to leave no doubt in anyone's mind that two courts, not just one, had declared Coke to be a wholesome harmless non-habit-forming beverage. Candler still could not understand the limitations and implications of the two verdicts.

The year 1912 might have been the least satisfying of Dr. Wiley's many years of government service. News of the trial's disappointing outcome was compounded by having to meet the bureau's obligation to cover court expenses of two hundred thousand dollars (five million in today's dollars). But the cost in terms of reputation and diminishing power to enforce the food and drug laws was incalculable. Wiley's requests for product seizures were now routinely denied. Secretary Wilson cited the bureau's dereliction of duty for paying little attention to a shameful patent drug industry while focusing almost exclusively on dubious food issues.

Wiley correctly perceived that his boss was looking for evidence to support firing him. Soon after the Chattanooga trial, an opportunity presented itself. The Bureau of Chemistry was accustomed to paying its experts a daily fee of $20. Dr. Henry Rusby, who had long served Wiley as an adviser, agreed to testify but demanded fifty dollars a day like the Coca-Cola experts sitting across the aisle from him. Wiley couldn't risk losing him so he concocted a scheme to provide Busby with a part-time government salary of sixteen hundred dollars a year. Rusby's limited work schedule achieved the desired hourly rate. Made aware of the deception, Wilson could now rid himself and the USDA of the troublesome chemist. An investigative panel was convened under Indiana Congressman Ralph Moss, thus assuring Wiley an opportunity to give voice to his side of the story. But the Moss committee also heard plenty of criticism from recognized authorities such as Ira Remsen, a noted food chemist who was also president of Johns Hopkins University. Although the panel exonerated Wiley of financial mischief, it demanded "a general reorganization of the bureau if the [food] law is ever to be effective."[67]

Wilson refused Wiley's demand for a change in oversight of his decisions, giving the chemist a basis for resignation. President Taft later distributed for public notice a "We're sorry to lose Dr. Wiley" memorandum that fooled no one. Editors of *Scientific American* took the occasion of Wiley's resignation to accuse him of maintaining an "Augean Stable filled with a thirty year accumulation of shoddy scientific thinking." They called for either a clean sweep of the bureau or repeal of what was termed the "Pure Foolishness Act of 1906."[68]

Even before his fate was determined, Wiley had considered a number of offers and accepted from *Good Housekeeping* the title editor-at-large. The popular magazine's publishers were so pleased to have Wiley they established him in a grand office with a magnificent view of Washington's Capitol district. For Wiley's irrepressible ego, this was a major step up from the cubicle he had long occupied at the USDA. From his perch, he wrote one polemic after another, many directed at his favorite target of all, the Coca-Cola Company.[69]

What had Dr. Wiley gained or lost for his agency during nearly three decades of public service? When he arrived in Washington, he epitomized a new standard of educational achievement and technical expertise. He was entirely committed to his mission: assuring for the American public the purest food supply that modern agriculture and the food industry could provide. Wiley worked tirelessly, even at the expense of his own personal life. He recognized early the need for federal legislation and was relentless in his pursuit of statutory authority. Unfortunately, his rigidly held convictions, many of them contrary to accepted science, got him in trouble. He was not even willing to bend in the face of a presidential rebuke. Yet he could always capture the support of the American people, most of them poorly informed about the scientific issues in question. Political leaders suspicious of Wiley were therefore unwilling to face him down for fear of losing the support of their electorate.

While it has been argued that the food bill would not have passed without Wiley's influence, it might have become law much sooner without the dissonance he created. As food law historian Peter Barton Hutt has argued, the circumstances leading to passage of the 1906 legislation fell into place regardless of Wiley's input; its time had come. "Wiley didn't make it happen by himself. Once the law was in force, Wiley contributed to its imprecision by taking positions unsupported by good science. His undoing was the Coca-Cola case, a skirmish that he could not pass up and blundered into without the evidence required for victory."[70]

The Coca-Cola case is detailed here because it serves as a template for similar actions taken by regulatory agencies over the course of a century, up to and including the FDA's assault on silicone breast implants: First, identify an alleged but unsubstantiated risk to consumers, and then follow with a product seizure. Gird for a battle that includes recruitment of opposing experts, and follow with a public spectacle, nowadays more often held in public hearing rooms with klieg lights and cameras than in a remote district courtroom. Furthermore, the plaintiff's bar presently stands prepared to initiate legal action as soon as any instrument of government so much as hints of a putative risk.

Not long after the 1911 trial in Chattanooga was ending, the bureau suffered another humiliating trial defeat. In *United States vs. Lexington Mill and Elevator*, the offending act was a bleaching process borrowed from the Irish. Nitrous peroxide was used to convert yellow spring and winter wheat into snowy-white flour that brought a higher market price but left a trace of nitrous acid residue. In Wiley's view it was adulteration of nature's bounty. Chemists speaking for the milling industry pointed out that ten thousand loaves of bread were needed for one medicinal dose of the nitrite. The bureau had failed to take into account a principle established in the sixteenth century by the Swiss physician Paracelsus: "Poison is everywhere . . . the dosage makes it a poison or a remedy." Although a district court jury ruled in favor of the government, an appellate court reversal was affirmed by the US Supreme Court, whose opinion stated the obvious: "government must establish a reasonable link between a substance and the alleged hazardous effect."[71]

The Moss committee's recommendation left no room for postponement; the Bureau of Chemistry had to clean up its act if the 1906 law was to serve as the nation's guarantor of food and drug safety. Prior to completing his sixteen-year cabinet term and accepting a distinguished academic post, Secretary Wilson tried but failed to attract an outside leader for the bureau, appointing instead a series of in-house replacements, most of them protégés of Wiley. None fulfilled Wilson's hope for decisive action against unscrupulous drugmakers.

Over the course of the next decade, the very existence of the Bureau of Chemistry would be challenged repeatedly as the government established new regulatory agencies. One of these, the Federal Trade Commission, believed that without the taint of so many courtroom defeats, it could more effectively fulfill the bureau's mandates. It very nearly succeeded.

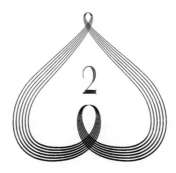

POLYMER CHAINS
AND WARTIME
MOBILIZATION

". . . an uninviting glue."
—Prof. Frederick Kipping, 1907[72]

"Now you've got something that I want . . . tomorrow!"
—Capt. Hyman Rickover USN, 1940[73]

While "Doc" Pemberton concocted his mildly addictive "French Wine Coca" and tested its kick on Atlanta's consumers, British chemist Frederick S. Kipping was committed to a career-long investigation of polymer chains, complex linear molecules that nowadays serve as the building blocks of fabrics, plastics, and pharmaceuticals, to name just a few. Unlike Pemberton, Kipping pursued the finest education available to him. Like Harvey Washington Wiley, he supplemented his science studies with research in Germany. Soon after returning to England, he was elected a Fellow of the Royal Society and appointed Chair of

Chemistry at University College Nottingham where he remained for the rest of his professional career.[74]

Professor Kipping became proficient at building complex linear chemical units. Unlike his colleagues who were more interested in familiar carbon-to-carbon chains, his fascination was with the binding nature of silicon, an element that makes up one quarter of the earth's crust. Unlike gold or mercury, silicon exists in nature only in combination with other elements like oxygen. One unit of silicon and two of oxygen makes silicon dioxide, a rigid molecule that exists in nature as sand, or when subjected to very high pressure, as quartz or granite. Applying polymerization technology, Kipping created a tightly bonded silicon-oxygen-silicon spine as durable as quartz. To this framework he attached various carbon-based groups that gave the chain a degree of flexibility never before seen by chemists. Among these compounds was polydimethylsiloxane or "silicone," a term he coined by fusing the words silicon and ketone.[75]

Swedish scientist Jons Jakob Berzelius was the first to isolate silicon, an element that had long resisted separation from naturally occurring compounds. He made another contribution that facilitated Kipping's research: showing that each compound of identical composition behaved differently according to its internal molecular architecture. Chains with identical chemical content he called "polymers." For example, starch, a simple polymer, is made up of multiple sugar units. Natural rubber, a more complex polymer, is constructed of isoprene units. As polymer chains were made longer, their physical properties changed. Kipping played these laboratory games for the remainder of his career.[76]

The noted polymer chemist lived and worked at a time when chemical discoveries were occurring faster than either the academy or industry could keep pace with. Between 1899 and 1944, Kipping published fifty-four articles in respected chemical journals, and as he continued to rearrange his polymer units, he loaded the shelves of his laboratory with beakers filled with cloudy viscous masses that annoyingly adhered to any surface they touched. He considered all of his "uninviting glues" to be useless. Kipping was less interested in the functional potential of his compounds than he was in defining laboratory conditions for their synthesis. Yet he recognized their resilience, especially the silicones; all of them were highly stable under extreme conditions. Their resistance to heat ranged from minus one hundred degrees to nine hundred degrees Fahrenheit. They were also resistant to most acids because of the silicon-oxygen-silicon backbone. With their various organic side chains, they were as malleable as rubber. Kipping eventually abandoned the silicones and moved on to other challenges. Not until the 1930s would the functional significance of these compounds receive their deserved recognition. In time, the professor's large family of organosilicon polymers would include solvents, lubricants, nonflammable hydraulic fluids, resins, high temperature seals, insulation, and the most remarkable biomaterials of the twentieth century.[77]

A young chemist, J. Franklin Hyde, rediscovered Kipping's work in the 1930s. After receiving his doctorate in chemistry, Hyde stunned his University of Illinois mentors by turning down a job offer from the esteemed DuPont Company where almost every bright young chemist wanted to work. Preferring independence from a large organization, he became the first organic chemist to join Corning, a glass-making company in upstate New York. It helped that his employers were willing to match DuPont's generous salary offer, $3,200 a year. The company's worry was the emergence of so many versatile polymers, some of them nearly transparent and thus competitive with glass products. What Corning's leaders needed for survival was the profitable exploitation of organosilicons. Specifically, they wanted as many commercial applications as Hyde's research could produce—and quickly. The young chemist's search of the scientific literature quickly revealed Kipping's work; it didn't take much more time for Hyde to recognize the career opportunity of a lifetime.[78]

His earliest laboratory efforts yielded the same nebulous materials that Kipping found so uninviting. But as the chemical reactions became more refined, the resulting products improved in quality and clarity according to chain length and cross-linkage.

They included liquids more fluid than water and others more viscous than oil, greases with the consistency of petroleum jelly, resins as hardened as varnish, and semi-solid blocks with the flexibility of rubber. Corning was asked by architects of the new Rockefeller Center to help fabricate an immense art glass window for the new RCA Building. Hyde selected organic polyvinyl acetate as his adhesive and with special permission from the glazier's union, positioned each of 240 polymer blocks himself. With increasing ease and production efficiency, the most appealing properties of organic polymers were merging with those of glass.[79]

Back in his Corning, New York, laboratory, Hyde worked on a silicone resin that displayed amazing resilience at extreme temperatures. Recognizing its potential for use as an insulating and lubricating grease in machinery operating at extreme conditions, he declared "990A" resin Corning's first patent-eligible product. While streamlining its production, Hyde received a visit from Hyman Rickover, a naval liaison officer assigned to the Electric Boat Division of the Bureau of Ships. What Rickover sought was an insulation material capable of withstanding the heat of a submarine's high performance engine and the frigid temperatures at the vessel's planned depth of operation. Hyde described the new resin's synthesis and properties in detail. "Now you've got something I want . . . tomorrow," Rickover exclaimed. The Navy had preauthorized him to place an immediate order; it was Corning's first commercial sale of a silicone product. Two hurdles remained. First, the synthetic process required magnesium, a scarce commodity reserved for aircraft production, and second, there was no facility large enough to produce the resin in quantities the military required. Rickover promptly secured the necessary magnesium priority, and Hyde asked for manufacturing assistance from the Dow Chemical Company of Midland, Michigan, coincidentally a major source of magnesium.[80]

Dow Chemical had previously mobilized for wartime chemical production during World War I, in time replacing Germany as the world's largest producer of phenols and aniline dyes. In 1941, President Roosevelt's War Production Board asked Dow to expand its extraction of magnesium from seawater in order to provide the tons required for accelerated aircraft production. Dow was already committed to the synthesis of chemical polymers, especially Styrene, an essential substitute for rubber production; Ethocel, a workhorse plastic used for goggles, canteens, waterproofing tents and combat clothing; and Saran, a versatile material that could be extruded into pipe and tubing, woven into fabric, or spread into thin sheets. After the war, Saran would become world famous as a food storage wrap.[81]

A $3 million pilot plant was built on land adjacent to the Dow Chemical complex with a production capacity of two hundred thousand pounds of 990A resin each month. In 1943, Dow Chemical and Corning Glass established a joint venture, Dow Corning Corporation, an enterprise that would endure long after completion of the war that prompted its creation. As the number of military applications for silicone polymers increased, production accelerated but quietly so; the existence of silicone remained classified throughout the conflict. Citizens of Midland didn't find out until 1946 that their community was growing at the rate of two expanding chemical companies, not just one.[82]

Word of the amazing new compounds spread quickly to all branches of the military. Early products included silicone fluid for dampening the vibrations in avionic equipment and a nonmelting grease for insulating spark plugs. Because petroleum lubricants turn to foam and bind engines operating above twenty thousand feet, Bendix Aviation selected Dow Corning 4 (DC4) as their most dependable lubricant. Ignition systems often shorted out at low altitudes over water, but the use of silicones virtually eliminated these power failures, permitting General Dwight Eisenhower to count on the faster P-47 Thunderbolt fighters for air cover during the North African landings. Prompt and safe flight of these aircraft across the Atlantic Ocean by way of South America saved the many weeks required for surface transport. Later in the war, silicone extended the range of B-17 Flying Fortresses on missions over Germany. Moreover, P-51 Mustang pursuit fighters could now accompany and protect those bombers from German interceptors, sparing the lives of hundreds of aircrews. Silicone seals, insulation, grease, and lubricants all contributed to safe flight of the B-29 Superfortress on its specialized missions over Japan at altitudes high enough to require pressurized cabins for the first time. Dow Corning scientists believed they had "produced the grease that helped win the war" and, indeed, they had. The unanticipated wartime success of organosilicon polymers prompted academic centers like MIT and the University of Pittsburgh's Mellon Institute to send their graduate students either to Corning or to Midland, where many were later employed.[83]

The most obvious advantage of the silicones was their thermal stability. Quite by accident, however, a precedent for clinical usefulness at normal temperatures was established near the end of the war. When medical corpsmen administered drugs such as morphine preloaded into glass syringes, a jammed syringe shattered easily. Paraffin coating was of limited help because syringes were more vulnerable after repeated sterilizations. Someone in the Army Medical Corps learned of a remarkable lubricant used by the aircraft mechanics. A tiny drop placed inside the chamber prior to sterilization was sufficient to eliminate the shattering glass problem. Medics were beginning to use a miraculous but scarce new drug, penicillin, for treating infections; elimination of syringe malfunction became essential. Because organosilicon polymers were chemically inert, they were assumed to be biologically inert also. Decades later, this assumption would be challenged in the courtroom.[84]

At war's end, demand for silicone nearly came to a halt. Military production requirements suddenly fell to less than 5 percent of the gigantic wartime output. Few strategists could imagine the forthcoming growth of commercial aviation, or the demands that the Cold War would place on military technological development. Instead, economists were forecasting a postwar decline in prosperity, similar to the recession that followed World War I. Despite these gloomy projections, unemployment in America remained low and aggregate spending in America began a climb that continued for two more decades. Domestic modernization and postponed infrastructure replacement helped to sustain full employment. Demand for consumer goods made scarce during the war was unprecedented. A wide variety of household appliances were paid for with accumulated military wages. The postwar baby boom served as its own economic stimulus. The devastation in Europe and other theaters of combat guaranteed years of demand for US agricultural products, manufactured goods, and construction assistance. Dow Corning executives wanted to participate fully in this rapidly expanding domestic economy so its research scientists were directed to "find something people will buy."[85]

The search for a versatile rubber substitute produced a resilient long chain polymer nicknamed "bouncing putty," later marketed for children as "Silly Putty." In time, silicone became an integral component of home insulation, water-resistant fabrics, all-weather caulking, glass coating, furniture polish and many more domestic products. Military applications were eventually adapted for postwar aerospace innovation and development.[86]

Tire production during the war required the forceful separation of synthetic rubber casts from a metallic mold that without an effective releasing wax yielded too many rejects. After silicone became the agent of choice, rejects were rare. The baking industry faced a similar challenge. Use of lard to free bread from pans created an acrid environment in most bakeries. A few drops of DC200 in each pan eliminated the use of lard forever. Originally marketed as "Pan Glaze," it cleared the air in commercial bakeries throughout the world.[87]

Taking their peacetime marching orders seriously, product developers came up with "SightSavers" for cleaning eyeglasses and "ShoeSavers" for all-weather protection of hiking boots and other leather products, new or used. Silicone rubber, trademarked as Silastic by Dow Corning, was fashioned into the "Gripmitt" for handling hot dishes. Brewers, vintners, and soft-drink bottlers, all faced with foaming problems during production, learned that a few drops of silicone added to their tanks reduced surface tension and eliminated the bubbles. Commercial sales of silicone products were taking off.[88]

Nearly all of these postwar applications involved direct human exposure to silicone polymers via skin contact or ingestion. Use of liquid silicones in cosmetic spray bottles and pressurized cans meant that microparticles could be inhaled. Dow Corning Director of Research Shailer Bass was concerned about the safety of his polymers, not because of reported incidents, but because silicone had never been studied for its toxic properties. Turning to corporate parent Dow Chemical and its toxicology laboratory, he asked for a comprehensive study of everything his company made. The results, published in 1948 by V. K. Rowe and associates, demonstrated that most silicone fluids were extremely well tolerated following subcutaneous and intraperitoneal injection, and essentially inert following inhalation or ingestion. Only the rarely used chlorosilanes, were found to be corrosive following vapor inhalation.[89]

In 1950, Bass visited the father of organosilicon chemistry at his seaside home in Wales. Retired from his academic post, Professor Kipping gratefully accepted a bound copy of his own published papers, along with subsequent publications from the Corning and Dow Corning laboratory groups. Kipping's personal records of scientific achievement had been destroyed during a wartime bombing raid. Bass tried to convince Kipping of the amazing diversity of modern silicone products. The old chemist listened but could recall only disappointment with his own amalgams."[90]

In a time of worldwide military conflict, a forgotten family of chemical polymers became essential for the success of innovative weapon systems with unprecedented performance requirements. Mankind has always responded to the pressures of war by inventing entirely new weapons. Without the stimulus of aerial and submarine combat and the subsequent introduction of myriad applications for the organosilicons, postwar society would have been a different place. Meanwhile, Dow Corning employees believed they were true pioneers, and they were.

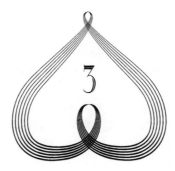

AN FDA VALIDATED
AND EMPOWERED

"The weak and the ailing furnish a fertile field for sale
of the unproven."
—Walter Campbell, FDA Commissioner, 1933[91]

When Shailer Bass asked Dow Chemical's toxicologists to define the limits of safety for silicone polymers, he was showing concern for the health and well-being of his staff. But he also knew that if the company wished to pursue medical applications for the silicones, strict regulatory standards would need to be met. Given a 1938 rewrite of the 1906 statute that included food, drugs, and cosmetics and some day the likelihood of medical devices, no manufacturer of eligible products could ignore the government's expanding oversight role. But empowerment of agencies like the FDA did not come easily.

Before the two world wars, the Bureau of Chemistry wasn't the only federal agency struggling for recognition and power. In 1914, the Clayton Act provided for a Bureau of Corporations empowered to investigate charges of unfair competitive practices by corporations large enough to engage in commerce across state borders. Soon enough, the agency recognized an opportunity to usurp the established regulatory functions of a weakened Bureau of Chemistry. With President Woodrow Wilson's backing and a congressional mandate, the Bureau of Corporations became the Federal Trade Commission, with power to impose significant fines. Not yet satisfied with its scope of influence, the FTC achieved a broader spectrum of responsibilities, among them oversight of advertising practices, but this brought it in conflict with the Department of Agriculture. Although the Bureau of Chemistry believed it was better qualified to deal with deceptive marketing of food and drugs, it had never established methods for postmarket monitoring of advertising practices. The assignment was soon lost to an opportunistic FTC.[92]

Because of the outcome of *United States vs. Coca-Cola*, a precise definition of "adulteration" and "misbranding" was in doubt, leaving the 1906 law without legal standing in a courtroom. Manufacturers large and small could hide behind their distinctive trademark name just as Coca-Cola had done. Department of Justice attorneys, believing that the pure food law deserved a rescue attempt, took the appellate ruling to the Supreme Court for review.[93]

On February 29, 1916, attorneys arguing for the federal government and the Coca-Cola Corporation appeared before Chief Justice Edward White and Associate Justices McKenna, Holmes, Day, Hughes, Devanter, Pitney, Brandeis, and Clarke. Representing Coca-Cola, Harold Hirsch argued once more that because the original formula contained no additives, it was beyond the court's jurisdiction. This time the justices weren't buying his logic. "If this were so," Justice Hughes later wrote, "manufacturers would be free to put arsenic into the original compound and sell the lethal mixture under a fanciful name."[94]

With respect to the misbranding, Hughes challenged Coca-Cola's distinctive name theory and offered a counter argument: "that given the court's agreement . . . a manufacturer could designate a mixture as 'Chocolate-Vanilla' even though it was destitute of either one or both ingredients, provided of course, that the combined name had not been previously used and thus qualified for trademark approval." The company's entire defense was essentially declared illegitimate: "By order of unanimity of the Justices of the Supreme Court the judgment is reversed and remanded [returned] for further review." Once again the court had sidestepped the question of caffeine's risk to consumers. But it had clearly reestablished the law's jurisdiction over food and drug products regardless of their formulation or trademark.[95]

The stunning news fell heavily on Coca-Cola executives in Atlanta for it meant the cloud of litigation would continue to hover over the Candler family enterprise. Dr. Wiley on the other hand was thrilled, and immediately wrote a victory column for *Good Housekeeping*. In it, he claimed total vindication, despite the fact that the popular beverage contained as much caffeine as it ever had. A mediated settlement seemed the only sensible way out. Unlike his father, Howard Candler was willing to compromise, agreeing to reduce the caffeine content of his beverage, a move that would force the bureau to file its case anew based on the revised formula. Nobody wanted that. Once again Coca-Cola had outsmarted the government. Soon thereafter, the company took back its forty barrels and twenty kegs of now rancid syrup concentrate.[96]

Why hadn't the parties in this case sought compromise earlier? Reducing the caffeine without damaging the flavor was always an option. Where was the benefit from these lengthy proceedings other than the empowerment of regulators and their adversaries? Similar questions would be raised when future prosecutors took on ATT, Microsoft, and Apple.

What at first appeared to be an astounding judicial victory for a beleaguered government bureau made little impact on its public image. Neither was any praise coming from the White

House. President Taft took note only of the government's many stumbling defeats. Throughout the 1920s, the bureau suffered repeated administrative setbacks and numerous leadership turnovers. A 1927 reorganization of the Department of Agriculture resulted in the renaming of bureaus and reshuffling of responsibilities. The Bureau of Chemistry's regulatory functions became the Food, Drug, and Insecticide Administration, while the laboratory and research mission was transferred to the Bureau of Soils. Three years later, the agency's name was abbreviated to Food and Drug Administration. In 1940 it was transferred to the newly formed Federal Security Agency (FSA), and then in 1953, was moved to the Department of Health, Education, and Welfare (DHEW), whose name would become the Department of Health and Human Services (DHHS) in 1980.[97]

Watching helplessly from his office at *Good Housekeeping*, Dr. Wiley could hardly control his rage when told that his cherished research laboratory belonged to the Bureau of Soils. He vented his anger in a 1929 polemic titled *The History of a Crime Against the Food Law*, 413 pages of uninterrupted rant. Regrettably, his life drew to a close just as the nation's next champion for more effective food and drug law, Franklin Delano Roosevelt, set in motion his campaign for the presidency. Wiley, a man of genuine dedication to government service, died in despair at his Northern Virginia farm in 1930.[98]

Few political contrasts in United States history were as stark as the two presidential candidates in 1932. Herbert Hoover, a man of simple Midwest origins with a record of extraordinary managerial achievement behind him, asked crooner Rudy Vallee to compose an antidepression campaign song. The result—"Brother, Can You Spare a Dime?"—failed to boost anyone's spirit as Hoover hoped it might. Roosevelt, a Northeastern patrician with no experience in the world of commerce, chose for his campaign's musical theme a lyric adapted from an MGM musical titled "Happy Days are Here Again!" It was an immediate hit and demonstrated to a desperate electorate that he was their man for troubled times. FDR inherited a nation in crisis, its economy in shambles, its banking system at the brink of collapse, its unemployment soaring, its populace despondent. Yet between March and June of 1933, he convinced Congress to enact fifteen major bills, plus found time to declare an immediate need for rewriting the original 1906 pure food legislation. "Let's give it some teeth."[99]

FDR was eager to show political continuity with his fifth cousin, Theodore. Although TR had listed food and drug oversight as one of his major achievements, the "Wiley Law" remained inadequate for dealing with countless abuses found in the marketplace. Statutory provisions were outdated with respect to existing public hazards. Government attorneys were forced to prove fraudulent intent in any case of alleged misbranding, always a difficult court challenge. The FDA held no controlling authority over false advertising, having lost that function to the FTC. Cosmetics were not even covered by the 1906 law. New products were coming to market daily without prior evaluation because premarket approval was never required for foods and drugs as it was for meat.[100]

FDR summoned the press on May 26, 1933, and announced he would welcome a new food and drug bill, strongly urging that it be considered during the fall term of Congress. New York senator and homeopathic physician Royal Copeland agreed to serve as principal sponsor. The Copeland bill became the Food, Drug, and Cosmetic Act of 1938 but not without fierce combat. Trade organizations and their lobbyists made clear they were prepared to fight as long as it took to defeat the measure.[101]

Meanwhile, the potency of new drugs was growing exponentially. A few compounds derived from aniline dyes were capable of inhibiting bacterial growth. The most effective of these was sulfanilamide, first studied by Leonard Colebrook of Queen Charlotte's Hospital London, who reported cures of streptococcal infections like puerperal fever. In 1936, Dr. Perrin Long of Johns Hopkins Hospital heard Colebrook present his clinical experience in London and brought the drug to Baltimore for additional testing. News of the miracle drug spread quickly. Late one evening, Long received a call from Eleanor Roosevelt; her infant son,

Franklin Jr., lay desperately ill in Boston and was not expected to survive a throat infection invading the bloodstream. Prontosil, the first commercial sulfa preparation, was rushed to the Massachusetts General Hospital, and news of the dramatic cure made the headlines. The *New York Times* contrasted the recovery of young Roosevelt with the tragic streptococcal death of President Coolidge's son ten years before.[102]

Licenses to produce the miracle drug cure were issued to several manufacturers, including the S. E. Massengill Company of Bristol, Tennessee. The company released sulfanilamide as an elixir in October 1937, ideal for children unwilling to swallow pills. Never a drug that suspended easily, Massengill's chemist, Harold Watkins, achieved success using diethylene glycol. After adding saccharin, caramel, amaranth, and raspberry extract, he tested for clarity, stability, and flavor on the tongue. Fortunately for professional tasters, swallowing was not required. Watkin's error was a momentary lapse of chemical memory; he had confused glycerols with glycols, the former well known for safe consumption, the latter an engine coolant toxic for all human use. For this error, Watkins would later end his personal torment by committing suicide.

Although the FDA has since claimed credit for spotting the chemist's error, it was the American Medical Association (AMA) Council on Pharmacy and Chemistry that took immediate action after receiving notice of trouble following use of the elixir. In the absence of effective drug oversight, the AMA had established its drug council in the 1890s for the benefit of physicians needing information about drug side effects. On October 11, 1937, two telegrams from Tulsa, Oklahoma, arrived at the AMA's Chicago headquarters. They announced six sudden unexplained deaths following ingestion of Elixir Sulfanilamide Massengill. The company had never asked for AMA approval of its new drug because there was no legal requirement to do so. Many ethical pharmaceutical manufacturers did seek a review of their products because AMA approval was good for business. Consultants quickly identified the solvent and conducted animal tests that confirmed the elixir's lethal potential for adults and especially for children. Morris Fishbein, editor of the *Journal of the American Medical Association (JAMA)*, stopped the Reuben Donnelley printing presses so that his October 28 issue could transmit a full accounting of the tragedy to the nation's physicians. No one could recall a similar drug catastrophe or a faster response from a professional organization—seventeen days.[103]

The FDA received notice of the Tulsa deaths on October 14, three days after the AMA learned of them, and sent inspectors to study the victims' medical records. Death in each case was acute kidney failure. Even before FDA inspectors arrived at his door, Sam Massengill knew he had a serious problem; nothing less than the company's entire fate was at risk. Yet he would never acknowledge diethylene glycol as the cause of death. Instead, he tried to shift blame to producers of the sulfa powder. Meanwhile staff members were on the phones around the clock or sending telegrams to prevent further tragedy.[104]

In Washington, Senator Copeland lost no time bringing news of the Elixir Sulfanilamide disaster to the attention of Congress. Resolutions were passed calling for an immediate accounting of the tragedy by Secretary of Agriculture Henry Wallace. On November 26, Wallace came to the Hill to reassure Congress that following quick action by the FDA, 228 of 240 gallons produced had been seized and destroyed. Because the 1906 law precluded seizures of drugs not yet proved dangerous, FDA officials had resorted to a charge of misbranding. The word elixir implied an alcohol-base, but the solvent in question was not alcohol, so misuse of the word elixir violated the law. FDA officials loved the story because the public learned just how weak the existing statute was. Meanwhile, committees produced new wording to assure the needed power. As the death toll mounted, there was little that trade association lobbyists could do or say.

In the end, 107 deaths were recorded from ingestion of Elixir Sulfanilamide Massengill, most of them children because streptococcus infects the young more than it afflicts adults. Twelve gallons of the preparation had been dispensed before the tragedy was revealed; only one was consumed. Then as now, patients didn't always take their medicine as directed. Someone calculated that if all 240 gallons had been swallowed, there might have been four thousand deaths. Secretary Wallace was correct: the FDA had acted decisively, but so had the Tulsa Medical Society, the American Medical Association, Reuben Donnelley Publishers, Western Union, even the S. E. Massengill Company. Yet it was as common in that day as it is today for a government official to avoid sharing credit with the private sector for duties that lie within that agency's jurisdiction.[105]

Despite intense pressure, another eight months passed between the sulfanilamide deaths and final action on the Copeland Bill. Letters from mothers of the victims were sent to the president pleading for the bill's passage. Women's organizations throughout the nation rallied in support of the strongest possible legislation. Secretary Wallace later testified that in order to prevent future disasters, the FDA must license every drug sold in the nation. Corporate lobbying intensified and legislators in both houses caved; licensing authority was considered too extreme. A proposal requiring on-site inspections was likened to Soviet-style police tactics. Even Senator Copeland disliked such radical measures, so his job was to find a compromise that all sides could accept.[106]

The Food, Drug, and Cosmetic Act of 1938 provided the FDA with greater control over the release of new drugs. Granted a new weapon, the court injunction, approval could be withheld if the company failed to prove a new drug safe. Labels with accurate warnings and precise directions for use were required. Only prescriptions written by physicians were exempted, the assumption being that doctors provided their own instructions. Thus a distinction was established between drugs requiring a prescription and drugs sold over the counter. For foods, new labeling standards were established and sanitary production conditions enforced. The new law was a gigantic leap for regulators.[107]

Cosmetics, a rapidly expanding business sector, were covered for the first time. Hair dyes, deodorants, antiperspirants, moisturizers, breath fresheners, wrinkle removers, hair restorers, rouge, even bust enhancing creams had been used since Roman times. Dr. Wiley's inspectors knew that commonly available hair depilatories were sufficiently inflammatory to leave permanent scarring. Section 701 of the 1938 Act called for public hearings to define acceptable standards. The first effective program for animal testing of cosmetics was initiated and later accepted by the industry.[108]

The FDA had hoped for greater control over unproven medical devices. In his 1933 annual report, FDA Commissioner Walter Crawford said, "the weak and ailing furnish a fertile field for the sale of unproven devices." He cited examples whose very names spoke for their ineffectiveness: the Reich Orgone Accumulator and the Hubbard Electropsychometer. Popular books like Morris Fishbein's *Fads and Quackery in Healing* and Richard Lamb's *American Chamber of Horrors* offered warnings against these contraptions. Senator Copeland reminded his colleagues there were countless faulty devices claiming to improve body function that deserved the same scrutiny as any medicinal product. But the 1938 Act limited the FDA's authority to adulteration or misbranding violations. Adulteration of a device was broadly defined as any variance from the function claimed; misbranding meant any unproven health claim. Labeling requirements included complete directions for use of the device and warnings against misuse. Because implantable devices were not yet a common feature of surgical practice, the law paid little attention to them.

The final skirmish was between the FDA and its traditional rival, the FTC; once again the issue was advertising oversight. Faced with the inevitability of a stronger law, industry lobbyists sided with the FTC because a cease-and-desist order was less condemning than a product seizure. And so the FTC prevailed once again. Their jurisdiction was assured by the Wheeler-Lea Act, a law that perpetuated the irrationality of one agency regulating claims made on a drug's label, while another agency regulated claims made in a newspaper, on the radio, or in time television screens. Wheeler-Lea remains in force to this day.[109]

The Federal Food, Drug, and Cosmetic Act was signed into law by President Roosevelt on June 25, 1938, a few days short of the 1906 law's thirty-second anniversary. Had Dr. Wiley lived to see the stronger law, he would have been jubilant. Also, he would have been pleased to learn from Commissioner Campbell that his favorite adversary, Coca-Cola, was under investigation once again. More sensitive testing had revealed traces of ecgonine, an obscure cocaine derivative. Forced to reveal the quantity of ecgonine at one part per fifty million, Campbell withdrew and Coca-Cola won a labeling exemption. Having to list cocaine or even one of its chemical relatives as an ingredient would have been a public relations disaster for the beverage maker.[110]

Given his new statutory power, Campbell no longer needed to engage in petty skirmishes of this kind. His agency faced administrative challenges beyond anything it had experienced in the past. Like the original law, the 1938 act was not self-enacting. Its real power would come from standards awaiting definition and regulations not yet written. The anticipated time for a full activation of the law was two years. That interval would be filled with hearings, consultant reports, written drafts, proposed revisions, and endless negotiations with trade representatives. Not one of these steps could be expected to proceed at optimum speed; deadlines were extended time and again. Nonetheless, government regulators believed the five-year struggle was well worth the effort and that American consumers were better off for the protections guaranteed.

The nation's pharmaceutical industry was coming of age in the 1930s, along with therapeutic efficacy of its latest products. The dominance of patent drug producers such as "Doc" Pemberton was a part of the past. Although scientists who left the academy for industry were often ridiculed and sometimes expelled from their professional organizations, George Merck almost single-handedly reversed this ingrained prejudice against corporate research. In 1933, he established a pharmaceutical research laboratory with a campus atmosphere and populated its well-equipped laboratories with the best scientists he could attract. Merck paid them well and granted them the greatest possible latitude and scope in pursuing their scientific goals. Other major drug firms with a matching vision adopted Merck's model. The impact of sulfa drugs on mortality from infectious disease inspired scientists to pursue projects of similar scope and influence. Despite a dismal outlook for the national economy, it was a time for optimism among chemists positioned to exploit molecular innovation.

The 1938 act served as a stimulus for scientists in corporate laboratories to conduct research according to the highest scientific standards. Both industry and the government realized that every new medicinal product would have to pass mutually determined requirements. For the first time, the conduct of meticulously designed clinical trials became essential for the necessary approvals. Few would ever again deny or resist the FDA's awesome power. Nonetheless, the agency's gathering momentum soon encountered obstacles of a different kind: limited resources in the face of an impending wartime economy. Drug regulators would not be able to impose the full power of their statutory mandate for another decade.[111]

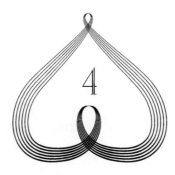

SILICONE AND A
PATIENT'S SELF-IMAGE

*"The three wishes of every man: to be healthy, to be rich
by honest means, and to be beautiful."*
—Plato

*"Beauty is a greater recommendation
than any letter of introduction."*
—Aristotle

L ike Mark Twain several decades before him, James Barrett
Brown grew up on the Mississippi River near Hannibal,
Missouri; he also knew something about transporting people over water. Appointed in 1941 as chief consultant in plastic
surgery for the European Theater of Military Operations, Brown's
challenge was transoceanic deployment of reconstructive surgical services for thousands of traumatically deformed combat
victims. Because ships departing American ports were filled to
capacity but returned nearly empty, it made better sense to bring
the wounded home to specialized centers staffed for long-term

rehabilitation than to send the needed personnel overseas. Brown proposed a timely evacuation of casualties to a fully staffed facility nearest home. The surgeon general accepted Brown's plan and authorized eight centers for reconstructive surgery, the largest of them at Valley Forge, Pennsylvania.[112]

While Colonel Brown directed more plastic and reconstructive surgeons than ever before assembled for a coordinated objective, he offered his own surgical talents to hundreds of casualties at the Valley Forge facility. Recognized as a pioneer in the care of burn injuries, he advocated early skin grafting for healing a burn. Recovery depended on the transfer of banked donor skin, a technique Brown perfected. Following termination of his wartime responsibilities, he returned to his prewar position as chief of plastic surgery at Barnes Hospital in St. Louis.[113]

Whether or not Brown was aware of silicone's numerous military applications, he was known to be vigilant for innovative surgical products. In 1947, a colleague called his attention to a remarkable new silicone fluid that was attracting interest for its protective affect on damaged skin surfaces. Brown thought it might ease suffering from burn injury, perhaps even facilitate the healing of skin graft donor sites. During a postwar visit to Dow Corning's Midland facilities, Brown studied the polymer in various physical formats that included custom carved flexible blocks useful for correcting facial defects following cancer surgery. After conducting animal experiments with silicone, Brown recognized the advantage of a synthetic product whose tissue compatibility was integral to its molecular structure. He reported his findings at meetings of plastic surgeons and correctly predicted that manufacturers would soon make a variety of silicone products available.[114]

The emerging silicone industry welcomed the interest of medical science, especially surgeons willing to collaborate with in-house engineers. Any reasonable inquiry brought a prompt reply. Requests for product samples were filled without charge but arrived with a request for timely feedback. Abdominal surgeon Frank Lahey, disappointed with his use of a rigid Vitallium tube for replacing damaged bile ducts, found that tissue-tolerant silicone tubing was ideal for his needs. Urological surgeon Robert De Nicola selected polyethylene tubing to repair a venereal stricture of the urethra but experienced better outcomes after switching to a silicone catheter.[115]

Another urologist, Robert Prentiss, reported successful use of Dow Corning's Silastic rubber for replacing congenitally missing testicles. Before WWII, artificial testicles were constructed using the metal Vitallium. Demand for these implants increased when disqualified recruits sought surgical replacement of a missing testicle. Following the war, Prentiss adopted a softer implant made of silicone gel.[116]

Pleas for help sometimes came from individuals faced with a personal crisis. John and Mary Holter feared the death of their child born with hydrocephalus, a potentially fatal birth defect. The brain is normally equipped with its own hydraulic pumping system that circulates fluid inside ventricles of the brain. Any obstruction to flow can lead to a buildup of fluid that compresses the brain. Holter, a hydraulic technician, was determined to save his child's life. Armed with facts provided by neurosurgeon Eugene Spitz, he attached a small valve to a polyethylene catheter only to find that blood soon clotted in the tubing. Substituting silicone tubing, the device remained open and kept cerebrospinal pressure within normal range. Not only was his child's life prolonged but many thousands of others have subsequently benefitted from the Holter Valve.[117]

Although Midland executives were pleased with the clinical success of their expanding medical product line, they faced a dilemma. The company's financial stability depended on steady revenue from patented products. Their research laboratory was continually distracted by one exciting new idea after another. Each new fabrication was made to specification without charge. Dow Corning couldn't even realize tax credits for its service to the medical community. In 1959, management established a tax-exempt corporate entity it called the Dow Corning Center for Aid to Medical Research. Its objective was to encourage physicians and engineers in their quest for new silicone applications. Silas A.

Braley became its executive secretary and served as liaison between the center and device innovators worldwide. Dow Corning executives did not yet employ medical professionals, so a monthly communication, *The Bulletin of the Dow Corning Center for Aid to Medical Research*, became the vehicle for widespread exchange of ideas. This unprecedented and hugely successful model could not possibly succeed today given the legal and regulatory environment in a society gripped by concerns about conflicts of interest, real and imagined.[118]

Within three years of Dow Corning establishing its research center, requests for silicone product exceeded the company's ability to satisfy demand. Market analysts recognized several promising commercial applications, among them silicone tubing of endless variety, intravascular catheters, and liquid polymers for syringe and needle lubrication. By 1962, conservative sales projections justified another bold step: formation of the Dow Corning Medical Products Division, a commitment that required capital investment and construction of another facility in nearby Hemlock, Michigan. A new American industry was under way, and its growth would be continuous for decades to come.[119]

Plastic surgeons have long been recognized and appreciated for their work with the physically deformed: children born with unwelcome birth defects, victims of burns and other trauma, and patients disfigured by cancer. But whenever the motive for surgery was improving natural appearance, the transaction became suspect. During the 1950s, only a few reconstructive surgeons were willing to care for patients seeking cosmetic surgery, and if so, they didn't talked much about it. The use of silicone for cosmetic applications wasn't due until the 1960s and the decades that followed.

Beauty as a basic desire of mankind is as old as recorded civilization itself. Asked why people coveted physical beauty, Aristotle replied, "No one who is not blind could ask that question." Archeological evidence confirms the use of cosmetics in Egypt four thousand years ago. Medieval women applied the blood of bats to their cheeks for enhancing their complexions. During the Renaissance, artists such as Albrecht Durer defined the proportions of an "ideal face," thereby influencing the representation of beauty in Western art for centuries to come.[120]

At the end of the nineteenth century, surgery remained a high-risk venture, especially when pursued for indications considered vain at the time. But this didn't restrain Charles Conrad Miller from surgically removing facial lines of expression, a forerunner of the modern facelift. Back in 1907, any surgeons willing to perform his procedure were ridiculed as a fringe element within their profession. But as the twentieth century evolved, a better understanding of the body's response to surgery yielded safeguards that allowed a patient to safely experience the stresses any surgery involves. Refinements in anesthesia eliminated any uncertainties of intentional loss of consciousness. Elective procedures to improve appearance involved so little risk that patients granted permission with increasing confidence. Nonetheless, the growth of cosmetic surgery continued to elicit resentment from a conservative medical profession.[121]

Even without formal training in the behavioral sciences, plastic surgeons learned from their patients how intense the motive for aesthetic surgery could be, especially when the body is subjected to the forces of pregnancy and aging. Twentieth-century culture assigns great importance to a youthful appearance. Body image is a recognized character trait, the conscious representation of an individual's appearance to others as well as to oneself. Personal well-being can depend as much on a person's self-image as it does on physical health. While some might think they can differentiate the motives for seeking reconstructive surgery from those for cosmetic surgery, the distinction is an elusive one. A patient seeking repair following removal of a facial skin cancer and another pondering a facelift are both dealing with related concerns.[122]

One reason that physical attractiveness can be dismissed as a valid psychological motive is that people assume few agree on who is attractive and who is not. But in practice, people can easily agree. In a landmark psychological study, subjects were asked to evaluate facial photographs, grade them for attractiveness, and then imagine characteristics like leadership, employability, and social desirability. Positive behaviors were assigned more often to the attractive images. But studies of this kind were suspect as long as they used college students as subjects. Psychologist Ellen Berscheid conducted similar studies using different populations in varied life settings. Nursery school children were shown pictures of adults and asked to say who looked kind and who appeared "scary." Retirees were asked to view pictures of children and rate them for popularity. Both young and old consistently preferred those they considered attractive. Within a hospital's newborn nursery, the cutest infants received more attention from the nursing staff. Mock jury studies demonstrated that physically unappealing defendants were judged guilty more frequently and received longer sentences. Despite life's varied predicaments, positive experiences correlate with eye-catching features. "Attractiveness is an important gift," mused philosopher Karl Popper.[123]

Plastic surgeons who took the time to inform themselves of these studies learned why their services were sought by so varied a population of patients. Furthermore, they realized the face was not the only feature in question. The same principles applied to the rest of the body, where certain definable proportions are considered more appealing than others. Premenopausal women taken to be healthy and attractive enjoy waist-to-hip ratios between .67 and .89. When photographs of Miss Americas from 1920–1980 were surveyed, their ratios (.69 to .72) were nearly identical to *Playboy* models: (.68 to .71). When hip and waist are placed in the context of another popular body parameter, breast size, the average supermodel measures 33–23–33 inches; *Playboy* models are only slightly larger. Even Twiggy, weighing just ninety-two pounds during her modeling prime and still remembered for her androgenous figure, measured a proportionate 31–24–33 inches, giving her a waist-to-hip ratio very close to the norm: .73. Although the person on the street is largely ignorant of numbers like these, both men and women can and do agree on which body contour they consider ideal.[124]

Wondering why men were so preoccupied with women's breasts, John Steinbeck wrote in *The Wayward Bus*, "A visitor from another planet might judge that the seat of procreation lay in the mammaries." A woman's breasts are like no others in the mammalian species; they take form at puberty and remain visible whether or not they are producing milk, whereas the breasts of other mammals enlarge only during pregnancy and become a sexual deterrent to their mates. In *The Naked Ape*, Desmond Morris theorizes that humans, after assuming an erect posture, developed rounded breasts as a way to transfer male interest to the frontal plane and encourage face-to-face bonding. Whether or not this explains the human mammary condition, it is clear to social anthropologists that men in most cultures admire the breast contours of youthful women.[125]

An obvious clue to the social importance of mammary glands is the anxiety the adolescent female experiences while waiting for breasts to develop. In modern society, teenagers generally make their own rules about what conforms and what does not. Clothing is always prominent on their list of desires but so is body shape, and in time, body function. Thelarche, the onset of breast development, can occur anytime between the ages of nine and sixteen, an event that is influenced by ethnicity, nutrition, and the hereditary precedent exhibited in a given family. The growth of the anatomic "mammary bud' is largely predetermined genetically but can be deterred by hormonal variations and on rare occasions by trauma; e.g., a severe burn. Developmental variations can range from the minimally visible to grotesquely overgrown, as well as breasts of unequal size. Although uncommon, one or both breasts may not develop at all. And so it should not be surprising that young women experiencing abnormal breast development often consult plastic surgeons. Some might delay for years, suffering embarrassment before summoning the courage.

Hugh Hefner, creative genius of Playboy Enterprises, is commonly held responsible for causing an exaggerated breast fixation during the 1950s. As he was reviewing proofs of a new magazine, Hefner acquired for five hundred dollars the nude photograph of actress Marilyn Monroe, who years before, had posed on a red velvet background, her shoulders rotated to feature both breasts. He sold fifty-three thousand copies of the inaugural issue, double the circulation hoped for, and they remain a collector's item today. While the belief that *Playboy* awakened an entire society's awareness of physical form is appealing, the notion overlooks historical precedent. Young men and old in the nineteenth century were titillated by catalogs whose pages displayed corsets and brassieres designed to accentuate a woman's breast profile and diminish her waist. On the pages of an 1897 Sears Roebuck and Company catalog were ads for bust creams specially compounded "for those whom nature has not favored."[126]

Surgery to replace a missing breast or to enlarge existing breasts dates from 1895 when Vincenz Czerny at the Academic Hospital of Heidelberg University published his account of the first reconstruction of a female breast. Well ahead of his time, Czerny maintained a strong interest in the transplantation of tissue. His restorations of nasal deformities with grafts of ear cartilage were the first of their kind. When a woman of the theater sought Czerny's advice about an expanding lump in her left breast, he took note of a coincidental fatty tumor (lipoma) in her flank. Because Czerny's patient was apprehensive of the asymmetry she might experience following removal of her breast tumor, he proposed transfer of the lipoma to restore the defect. According to Czerny, the fat graft afforded his patient with a "left breast that was well shaped and similar to the right." Today, we know that the fate of a free fat graft is limited by the dimensions of the tissue transferred. Czerny's graft was probably too large for complete survival. Six months later, using uncommon surgical candor, he admitted that his patient's breast was "somewhat smaller than desired."[127]

Czerny had been a student of Theodor Billroth, one of Europe's greatest surgeons, so his reputation was not jeopardized by efforts to restore normal body contour. But other surgeons who adopted the fat graft method for enlarging breasts were scorned by their colleagues, as were those who used unnatural materials for breast enlargement. Gersuny, in 1899, injected paraffin into the breasts, while others used vegetable oils, beeswax, lanolin, even glass beads for what was believed at the time a dubious surgical endeavor. For victims of breast cancer, neither injections nor fat grafting was appropriate because the surgical standard of the day was radical mastectomy, meaning removal of the entire breast and repairing the defect with grafts of skin. Flaps of adjacent skin could be rotated into the defect but the outcome was no less unsightly. Not until later in the century were methods devised for a more aesthetic restoration of breasts lost to cancer treatment.[128]

Silicone was only one of several postwar synthetic polymers. Entirely new industries emerged as a direct result of polymer innovations, among them moldable plastics. Unlike silicone, none of the new plastics enjoyed the same compatibility with human tissue. Nonetheless, at least four plastic polymers were fabricated in a sponge format applicable for cosmetic breast enlargement. In 1954, Pangman and Wallace reported five hundred successful augmentations using Ivalon. Neuman documented similar benefits from Polistan. Paula Regnault found success with Etheron. Least satisfactory was the use of Hydron. Yet none of these materials withstood the test of time because of a common failing: an open porous structure permitting absorption of protein-rich plasma that would soon clot and produce a rock-hard breast.[129]

Despite the outcomes, requests for implant removal were rare. Patients remained delighted with their contour improvement and accepted what could only be classified as an unsuitable texture. And so it became clear that a better mammary implant was needed, and two Houston plastic surgeons responded to the challenge: Thomas Cronin and Frank Gerow.[130]

Cronin, whose calm demeanor was more typical of a Midwest schoolmaster than a brassy Texan, always chose his words carefully and never raised his voice. At national conferences, the room would suddenly fall silent whenever he approached the microphone. No one present wanted to miss a single word of the wisdom he was famous for. "Cronin from Houston" he always began, even though everyone in the hall knew exactly who he was and what he represented: consummate surgical judgment. The techniques that he and his longstanding partner, Raymond Brauer, had perfected for the care of children with cleft lip and palate remain useful today. Referred to lovingly as "Big Daddy" by the resident surgeons he trained, Cronin always appeared to be deep in thought about surgical problems that awaited solution. For example, he had never been impressed by synthetic sponge breast implants and their stony fate. He recalled patients telling him they no longer danced socially out of fear that partners might learn of their breast surgery. Surely, he thought, there ought to be a more suitable material for the purpose.[131]

Frank Gerow, a resident-in-training at Houston's Baylor University Medical Center, was enthralled by his chief and the opportunity to work with him. Cronin recognized in Gerow a remarkably creative young surgeon, always willing to discuss problems and imagine creative solutions. One of Cronin's prior residents, Thomas Cresswell, practiced in Saginaw, Michigan, and sent news of a remarkable new polymer that Dow Corning was producing nearby. Already aware of silicone from Brown's reported experience with it, Cronin and Gerow pondered how they might use the material. While temporarily assigned to Baylor's affiliated Jefferson Davis Hospital, Gerow dealt with a frequent hospital problem: bedsores. He imagined a softer bed surface, one filled with a flexible material like silicone to reduce the pressure that led to bedsores. He also suggested liquid silicone immersion to facilitate wound healing. Dr. Melvin Spira later adapted the immersion method for treatment of burned hands.

In the meantime Cronin was persuaded that silicone might serve as the material he sought for breast surgery. Writing to Silas Braley at Dow Corning's Center for Aid to Medical Research early in January, 1961, Cronin described his own and Gerow's ideas and enclosed a wish list of materials he needed for experiments: eight ounces of liquid silicone, two to four ounces of Dow Corning adhesive, and three to four sheets of the elastomer that Dow Corning previously trademarked as Silastic. Cronin also asked if Dr. Gerow might visit the Midland facility and familiarize himself with the handling of these products.[132]

A prompt reply came from staff associate Ethel Mullison, who affirmed Dow Corning's interest in pursuing all the ideas proposed. She enclosed a copy of the toxicology studies performed by Dr. Rowe at Dow Chemical but discouraged Dr. Cronin's imagined use of a Silastic bag filled with liquid silicone for breast enlargement, explaining that membranes were permeable and silicone droplets could be expected to "leech from the bag." Instead, she urged Cronin to wait for an anticipated product with gel properties. Mullison welcomed a visit from Dr. Gerow who wasted little time making his way to Midland.[133]

Arriving on February 6, 1961, Gerow met Silas Braley and proceeded to work with the research staff from dawn to dusk. After three days, Gerow departed, carrying samples of everything he and his mentor had wanted and more . . . but not the new silicone gel just yet. Braley explained it would be forwarded at a later date. Cronin and Gerow began with animal experiments similar to those previously conducted by Dr. Brown in St. Louis. In time, they selected patients for use of carved Silastic for restoration of nasal contour defects. Cronin tailored thin sheets of the material for reconstructing the delicate orbital floor, and he also fashioned what he called an "armature" for restoring congenitally deformed ears. Silicone was proving to be more versatile in their hands than any prior synthetic material. For each application, the body accepted the implant without noticeable reaction.[134]

Before them lay their next challenge: design and fabrication of a mammary device. While in Midland, Gerow was shown samples of the gel format in development, a viscous derivative of room-temperature vulcanizing silicone. He initially thought of injecting the material directly behind the glandular breast but later abandoned that idea in favor of a self-contained device. Several more months of collaboration resolved questions about ideal size and shape, whether the volume should be adjustable, and how best to maintain the devices in position. A prototype model was filled with saline, but valve failures led to frequent deflations. A

Dacron patch was affixed to the under surface for promoting tissue adhesion and preventing the implant from moving. On January 24, 1962, Silas Braley informed Cronin that a gel device conforming to the latest design was ready, a prefilled and sealed mammary implant. Cronin accepted delivery in February and the first patient was selected.

Timmie Jean had initially consulted Dr. Gerow for removal of tattoos from each of her breasts; she disliked what they symbolized—a hardscrabble life. Married at 15 and divorced at 30 with six children, she described her breasts as "size 34 flat." "The doctors just looked at me and thought I was the perfect candidate. Why not, I thought." Timmie Jean received the first pair of Dow Corning mammary implants designated for clinical use in March 1962. Given the opportunity to see and touch the implants before her anesthetic, she declined. "Out of sight, out of mind," she later told a reporter. Following surgery, her chest "felt like a ton of bricks were lying on it." But she was a full C cup, just as her doctors had promised. "Boy, things began to look up after that," she exclaimed. By the following New Year's Eve, she was a remarried woman, Timmie Jean Lindsey, and ready for a different kind of life.[135]

At that time, breast implants did not arrive in Houston presterilized. Dr. Cronin's residents were assigned the task of preparing each device for implantation. Because of a residual layer of sticky gel adhering to the shell, they had to be scrubbed in detergent, then soaked in a soapy solution, and finally boiled and rinsed while they were still hot. Unwilling to hang around the hospital at the end of a busy surgical day for what amounted to a housekeeping chore, residents brought the devices home, where the responsibility was delegated to their wives. The next morning, the implants were brought back to the operating room, wrapped, and sterilized in an autoclave.[136]

Cronin withheld the news from Dow Corning until April 11 when he was convinced the result was superior to anything he had previously seen: "The first composite, natural-feel, Silastic breast prostheses have now been in place for three or four weeks," he wrote to Braley, enclosing photographs of the outcome but with apology for the tattoo removal scars. "She was one of Dr. Gerow's patients at the City-County Hospital and not one of my own."[137]

News spread rapidly among plastic surgeons in Houston and nearby cities as well. Dow Corning had agreed to withhold distribution of the devices until Cronin declared them safe for use. All implants were filled and sealed at Midland in sizes initially ranging from 230 cc to 270 cc. As the months passed, many more patients were implanted. On January 10, 1963, Cronin heard from Medical Products Division Manager William Rhodes, who was understandably eager to establish commercial availability of the devices for many more surgeons. Rhodes wanted to know whether patients were paying for their procedure; if so, then a charge for the device seemed appropriate. Cronin assured him that every patient thus far had received their devices on an experimental basis and were not expected to pay for the implants. Asked what price Dow Corning thought their device should bring in the marketplace, Rhodes' estimate was sixty to one hundred dollars a pair. Only then was the subject of royalties discussed for the first time.

The two Houston innovators decided to present their invention and their cumulative experience at a forthcoming International Congress of Plastic Surgeons in Washington, DC. Cronin would present the mammary implant data and Gerow his experience with silicone fluid immersion therapy. Meanwhile, Cronin attended an April 1963 meeting of plastic surgeons in Mexico City, where he couldn't resist offering a preview of his recent success. Writing to Silas Braley afterward, he reported an overwhelming response from his colleagues: "There exists a market which is hungrily awaiting these devices and I hope that you will be able to make delivery immediately." At the time, Dow Corning was preparing for an inaugural display of its new "Silastic Mammary Prosthesis" at the Washington congress. Meanwhile, the company was receiving "urgent" orders from plastic surgeons throughout the nation. Cronin agreed the time had come for commercial distribution but asked if he might compose instructions for his colleagues to follow. His document represented the first

Before   *After*

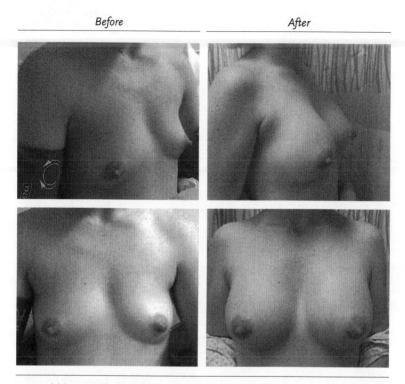

34 yr. old housewife with bilateral breast hypoplasia before and after bilateral breast augmentation. CREDIT: Anne Wallace MD

Before   *After*

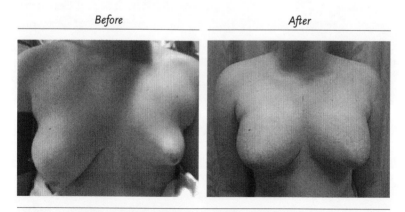

17 yr. old student with left breast hypoplasia, a developmental error, before and after right mastopexy (breast elevation) and bilateral implants for symmetry. CREDIT: Anne Wallace MD

product information data sheet that would thereafter accompany every implant distributed by Dow Corning. By August of 1963, twenty-five pairs of implants were shipped to nineteen surgeons along with a request for clinical feedback.

Years later, serious questions would be raised in courts of law regarding the adequacy of clinical testing for these devices. Trial attorneys would overlook the toxicology studies performed by Dow Chemical in 1948, and they would ignore all experiments conducted first by Brown and later by Cronin and Gerow. Lawyers would maintain that clinical trials had been omitted in order to accelerate commercial exploitation. How valid are these arguments?

The government's regulatory jurisdiction over medical devices, according to the 1938 rewriting of the food and drug law, was limited to "adulteration" and "misbranding." Cronin's mammary device was composed of two polymers already well known to the FDA: silicone and Dacron. Although production of the gel represented a new physical format, there was no chemical adulteration of either component. Neither was misbranding an issue; the declared purpose of the device was clear to surgeons and patients alike. Furthermore, directions for use and warnings based on the experience of several patients were provided by Dow Corning to every plastic surgeon electing to use the device. As for clinical trials, the term did not have the same meaning then that it has today. Cronin's personal oversight of the project, together with the clinical experience of several carefully selected surgeons, represented in 1963 as thorough a premarket trial of a medical device as had ever been conducted.

In Washington, Cronin presented his breast implant experience to an international audience gathered at the Shoreham Hotel. Not every plastic surgeon attending was interested in breast enlargement surgery, but when Cronin rose to speak in the grand ballroom, there was standing room only. The silicone polymers represented a new high standard for biocompatibility. The clinical results drew immediate praise, voiced even by surgeons from nations where silicone products were as yet unknown. Dow

Corning representatives exhibiting their product were kept busy with orders just as Cronin had recently predicted.

Nobody in 1963 challenged the validity of the product's development. Silicone gel mammary implants gained acceptance as quickly as demand for the sponge devices vanished. No one imagined that a day would come when blame was laid upon silicone for serving as a human carcinogen.[138]

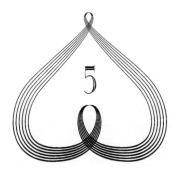

CONGRESSMAN DELANEY AND THE CANCER SCARE

*"Carcinogens are subtle, stealthy, sinister saboteurs of life.
They have no place in the food chain."*
—Congressman James J. Delaney, 1958

During the years of relative peace immediately following the Second World War, menaces still loomed in the minds of legislators inclined to conduct special investigations and write laws they believed necessary for the public's safety. Fearing an assault on American democratic ideals, Congress enacted the McCarren Internal Security Act, an anticommunist statute that in practice actually served to abridge individual rights. Consumed by his own belief in a traitorous government, Wisconsin Senator Joseph McCarthy forced a frenzied search for communists. Responding to the public's fear of widespread organized crime in America, Tennessee Senator Estes Kefauver achieved television fame and a vice-presidential nomination for his conduct of public hearings considered sensational at the time. Grief-stricken by his wife's unexplained intestinal malignancy, Brooklyn Congressman James J. Delaney was vulnerable to reports of an alleged cancer epidemic. No satisfactory explanation made sense to him other than the many new chemicals added to the food supply. Without any formal science education to his credit or any validation of his theories, Delaney convinced enough of his colleagues that the nation faced an impending cancer crisis, one that could be averted only by appointing a special committee to establish statutory limits on use of his perceived toxins. More recently referred to as chemophobia, the notion of widespread environmental poisoning still dominates our society's belief system.[139]

Appointed in 1950 as chairman of the House Select Committee to Investigate the Use of Chemicals in Foods and Cosmetics, Delaney worked tirelessly to inflame the public's fear of pesticides and additives, leading to the 1958 enactment of an empowering amendment to the Food, Drug, and Cosmetic Act. Among its provisions was a clause stipulating that no food additive shall be deemed safe if found to induce cancer when ingested by man *or animal*. Thereafter referred to as "The Delaney Clause," his mandate was enthusiastically embraced by consumer activists and environmentalists alike. Its language and impact would be reviled by industry as well as ridiculed by the scientific community for another four decades. Meanwhile, government bureaus such as the Environmental Protection Agency (EPA) sought to expand the scope of the law's restrictions, while the FDA was stuck with enforcing a statute it knew was scientifically indefensible.

In placing such unreasonable limits on food science, pharmaceutical innovation, and pesticide development, Delaney and his colleagues had ignored recognized principles of comparative physiology by assuming that all animal species respond the same to any and all carcinogens. Not until 1996 would Congress revisit the legislation, and vote unanimously for the Food Quality Protection Act that eliminated the zero tolerance limits on pesticides. Long before this reversal of statutory sentiment, the remarkable polymer that revealed so many unique properties in time of war and later in peacetime, polydimethylsiloxane, was added to the list of chemical compounds believed responsible for the putative cancer epidemic.[140]

News of the crisis came to most Americans in the form of newspaper and newsreel headlines announcing that cancer deaths had increased sharply since the beginning of the century. In 1900, malignancies were the eighth-leading cause of death in the United States, representing less than 4 percent of all human mortality in America. By 1945, the percentage of deaths from cancer had more than doubled, and by the end of the century, it was expected to reach 23 percent. Moreover, news editors often featured reports of so-called "cluster outbreaks," single communities experiencing an unusual number of cancers within a limited time interval. Then as now, such occurrences prompted wild speculation about presumed causes. Whenever a possible toxic source could be identified, the public customarily jumped to erroneous conclusions. A notorious example took place in Niagara Falls, New York, where the Hooker Chemical Company had deposited chemical effluent in and around the Love Canal throughout the 1940s and 1950s. After discovery, nearly every medical ailment experienced by local residents was attributed to chemical exposure, among them miscarriages, birth defects and of course cancer. Not just one cancer but any kind of cancer. Not one of these associations was ever confirmed, yet twenty-five hundred residents were relocated at a cost of thirty million dollars.[141]

What journalists and legislators weren't considering is that the population was not only growing but also living longer, twice as long since 1900. Except for rare cases of infant malignancies, cancer is a disease that occurs in the elderly. People have to live long enough to be vulnerable to a malignancy (76 percent of all cancers are diagnosed beyond 55 years of age). Most popular reports of an increase in the frequency of cancer lacked a statistical correction for the median age of subjects under study. Because more employers were providing health insurance, many more people were visiting their doctors regularly, which meant greater opportunity to detect a cancer. And because overall mortality is 100 percent, the ranking of any one cause of death is codependent on all the others. So the fact that cancer represented 4 percent of deaths in 1900 and 12 percent by 1950 is largely explained by a decrease in deaths from contagious disease. When all the mathematical corrections were made for population growth, life span, and other causes of death, there had been no increase in cancer mortality since 1900.[142]

Nevertheless, it was easy for people to believe that their risk of death from cancer was increasing. Visits to the doctor more commonly led to breast exams, mammograms, and biopsies of suspicious lumps. During pelvic examination, women were screened for cervical cancer by using the Papanicolaou cytologic staining technique, discovered in 1928 but not widely practiced until after WWII. Bleeding from the rectum led to a sigmoidoscopic examination and earlier diagnosis of bowel cancer. Skin cancers such as melanoma were reclassified to encourage earlier detection. All these measures meant more cancers revealed and treated earlier. As for widely publicized cancer cluster outbreaks, they were as difficult to interpret then as they are today. Toxic exposures rarely cause more than one malignancy, but affected communities usually experienced a medley of cancers and blamed them all on the accused toxin.[143]

Attitudes about cancer also changed following the war. A Roper Center for Public Opinion Research poll taken in 1945 revealed that 70 percent of people believed that tuberculosis, infantile paralysis, and syphilis represented their most serious health risks. Less than 30 percent listed cancer. Yet by the mid-1950s, public perceptions of risk had reversed, in part because of an increased fear of cancer.[144]

Only tobacco-related cancers of the lung were increasing in both incidence (new cases) and prevalence (existing cases). Because tobacco use had escalated since the 1930s, deaths from lung cancer were also rising. Any valid assessment of cancer mortality in America required that tobacco-induced cancer be considered independent of all other malignancies. Because the surgeon general did not issue his warning until 1964, the link between tobacco and cancer had not yet been taken into account, so Delaney's committee would hear only one theme: the growing danger of modern chemistry.

Many distinguished scientists attended the opening day of hearings, each of them willing to return and provide testimony. They came from academia, from private industry, and from selected government laboratories. Their fields of expertise included physiology, chemistry, nutrition, pharmacology, medicine, agronomy, entomology, and animal husbandry. Also present were executives from the baking, canning, meatpacking, and insecticide industries. Consumer organizations sent their representatives, as did the Federation of Women's Clubs. Among the science luminaries was University of Illinois Professor Andrew C. Ivy, who after winning a Nobel Prize in Medicine would in the declining years of his life achieve notoriety for promoting an unproven cancer cure-all.[145]

FDA Commissioner Paul Dunbar led off with a story calculated to place his agency in the most favorable light: a retelling of the elixir sulfanilamide saga that highlighted his dedicated inspectors' search for every last bottle of the poisonous syrup. He warned that the 1938 food and drug law held no provision for notification or testing of new chemicals added to food products. Acknowledging a need for the use of chemicals in the food supply, he shocked the committee with a listing of 842 known additives, 704 in current use, yet only 428 tested for safety. Agreeing that the safety of new additives ought to be proved in advance, Dunbar provided no indication that his agency could meet the challenge. When scientific experts were later queried about which government laboratories were equipped for advance testing, support for the FDA was found lacking.[146]

Later the panel heard testimony from Dr. John R. Matchett, a USDA chemist who admitted that his bureau's mission was to assist food producers with their development of chemical additives. Without enhanced flavors and consistent food textures, he added, there would be fewer packaged foods in neighborhood markets. To prove his point, he offered an unfortunate choice, the fourteen million dollar maraschino-cherry industry. The cherry in a Manhattan cocktail, he explained, was first stripped of its natural color using sulfur dioxide, then given its familiar scarlet color with an aniline dye. When a puzzled committee member asked why, Matchett blamed nature's unpredictable coloring and the consumer's demand for consistency. It didn't sell very well. Undeterred, he vouched for disodium phosphate as a necessary addition to evaporated milk products. Had Dr. Wiley been sitting in the gallery, he would have been horrified to learn his former bureau was a willing accomplice of an errant food industry.[147]

Although the Delaney hearings included no proud moments for agencies competing for jurisdiction, they did permit industry spokesmen to rebut evidence offered by government witnesses. Dr. Dunbar had accused monochloroacetic acid of being as toxic to humans as bichloride of mercury; Dr. Matchett had never heard of the compound. In rebuttal, Dr. Franklin C. Bing testified on behalf of the Council on Foods and Nutrition of the American Medical Association, citing pharmacological evidence that the preservative was harmless at dilutions commonly used by food processors. Bing explained that the threshold between safe and unsafe was determined by dosage. It was the Paracelsus principle given voice over again—the poison is in the dose—but it fell on deaf ears. Even today, harbingers of toxic doom still ignore the importance of dose response relationships when defining risk.[148]

The House Select Committee to Investigate Chemicals in Foods met for one last time on June 19, 1951. Congressman Delaney charged his staff with the task of collating 1,460 pages of testimony and issuing a report by January 1952. Their publication was remarkably free of the inflammatory language offered at hearings, for example, no charges thrown at food processors for "poisoning the American public." Committee members agreed there was need for only a few chemicals in processed foods. What the committee really wanted was the same premarket notification provision that the 1938 law required for new drugs. But congressional reports mean nothing without subsequent legislative action.[149]

One benefit of the investigation was a National Academy of Sciences (NAS) review of chemical additives in foods. Its report concluded that substances added to foods usually come from natural sources used for centuries, not from someone unmindful of public health. Nearly six hundred chemical additives were generally considered safe for human consumption. Despite reassurance from one of the nation's most respected advisory councils, Congress was determined to pass new legislation and it came in three parts: the Pesticide Amendment of 1954, the Food Additives Amendment of 1958, and the Color Additive Amendment of 1960. The best of the 1958 amendment was acceptance of the list of additives generally regarded as safe (GRAS); the worst was assigning to the FDA exclusive control over approving new additives. What followed were years of endless debates over the comparative risks and merits of artificial sweeteners like cyclamates and fat substitutes like Olestra.[150]

At no time during their deliberations did Congressman Delaney and his colleagues change their minds about more Americans dying of cancer. They never consulted scientists at NIH, one of whose institutes is entirely devoted to cancer. Its Epidemiology Branch operates the Surveillance, Epidemiology, and End Results (SEER) Program, an ambitious data-gathering enterprise. Neither did they consult with the tumor registries supported by states such as Connecticut, Iowa, New Mexico, Utah, and California. Instead, Delaney got what he originally wanted, a law stipulating that "no additive shall be deemed to be safe if it is found to induce cancer when ingested by man or animal."[151]

Despite resistance from the scientific community, Delaney was savvy enough to know that the public's reaction to his clause would be enthusiastic, and it was. In words carefully chosen for their impact, he announced: "Carcinogens are subtle, stealthy, sinister saboteurs of life. They have no place in our food chain." And so it was done.[152]

There is a reason for the ease with which tumors are produced in a laboratory mouse. These rodent strains are the product of deliberate genetic manipulation. Traits considered favorable for the laboratory are easily bred into the species: optimum litter size, predictable life span, dietary tolerance, infection resistance, and for certain strains, susceptibility to developing tumors. C. C. Little, a Harvard biology student in 1909, defied faculty opposition to what was disparaged as a "forced incest experiment" and pursued his objective, genetically identical offspring following twenty successive brother-sister matings. He called them isogenic or inbred mice. Throughout a distinguished career at the Roscoe B. Jackson Memorial Laboratory in Bar Harbor, Maine, Little produced many similar strains and was actually surprised to find they were susceptible to chemical carcinogens. Some new strains displayed as much as a 90 percent tumor occurrence rate. Rodent species living in nature according to the evolutionary laws of natural selection are not similarly vulnerable to cancer. While it should not have taken a person trained in tumor biology to realize that mice at special risk for cancer are not appropriate subjects for screening potential carcinogens, a few scientists and most legislators failed to realize that a tactical error was in play.[153]

Dr. Bruce Ames, professor of biochemistry and molecular biology at the University of California–Berkeley, is as qualified as any scientist to pass judgment on the validity of methods for determining any chemical's carcinogenic potential. Writer John Tierney once observed that "he has a quiet, kindly tone of authority as he patiently explains why things are the way they are." As creator of the Ames Test, which allows scientists to test chemical compounds for their ability to produce cell mutations that yield a cancer, his testimony at regulatory hearings often led to the banning of certain synthetic chemicals. A time came, however, when Ames changed his mind—a scientist's imperative whenever new evidence reveals itself. What alerted his doubt was the accepted experimental model for carcinogen testing: administration of a maximum tolerated dose (MTD) to susceptible laboratory animals over the span of two years, nearly a rodent's lifetime. But there wasn't anything natural about a maximum dose regimen [recall the government's laughable evidence in 1911 showing that rats fared poorly on a diet restricted to Coca-Cola syrup]. Also dubious was the assumption that synthetic chemicals were more likely to induce cancer than naturally occurring compounds. Ames knew that chemicals in both categories were capable of producing malignancies in the laboratory. In fact, the cumulative experience of cancer testing laboratories demonstrated that more than half of all natural and synthetic compounds are carcinogenic under the doubtful conditions adopted by government agencies.[154]

In the past, analytical laboratories were not capable of detecting small quantities of chemical compounds, but with improvements in technology, products from any garden, organic included, were found to contain carcinogens in trace amounts, parts per million or a billion in fact. A widely noted public information campaign sponsored by the American Council for Science and Health features a traditional Thanksgiving menu "laced with carcinogens," meaning naturally occurring chemicals falsely assumed to be lethal. They include aflatoxin in the mixed nuts, methyl eugenol in the salad, malonaldehyde in the roasted free-range turkey, acrylamide in the bread stuffing, furan derivatives in the cranberry sauce, and benzapyrene in homemade pumpkin pie. None of these are present in more than trace quantities, and the testing that found each chemical to be carcinogenic was based on the lifetime MTD model. For Thanksgiving gourmands to achieve the mouse carcinogenic dose of malonaldehyde, for example, they would need to consume 3.8 tons of turkey, quickly![155]

Ames was not alone among scientists when he reasoned that the ease of producing experimental tumors failed to correlate with reasonable human exposures to ordinary foods. Nonetheless, the wording of the Delaney Clause left no wiggle room, no exceptions, no option for adaptive reasoning. When a government agency wants to define regulations without interpretive flexibility, it can do so if Congress assigns the authority. That is what the FDA proceeded to do, along with the Environmental Protection Agency, the Occupational Safety and Health Administration, and the Consumer Product Safety Commission. Notably missing was the National Cancer Institute, this nation's federal authority best qualified to define causes of *human* cancer.[156]

Based on his own evidence, Ames transferred his intellectual support to the other side of the chemical-ban debate, declaring that natural carcinogens were pervasive in our food supply, at our work sites, throughout our environment, yet produced no grave consequences. Together with his UC–Berkeley collaborator, Lois Gold, his experiments established that human diets will never be free of naturally occurring carcinogens. What Ames was trying to discourage was the false presumption of hazard from trace exposures to chemical compounds, including pesticides. But like a changeling who suddenly sings a different tune, Ames encountered abuse from all four government agencies committed to the stipulated carcinogen testing model. He was experiencing first-hand the conflict between science and the politics of risk.[157]

"Even a naturally grown coffee bean is filled with chemicals," he told writer Virginia Postrel. "They've identified more than a thousand . . . but we only found twenty-two that have been tested in animals and seventeen of those are carcinogens. There are more than ten milligrams of known carcinogens in every cup of coffee," he added, "and that is far more than you'll likely receive from pesticide residues in an entire year." While the FDA could not effectively restrict the drinking of coffee, it could go after what people put in their coffee and it did. Artificial sweeteners such as saccharine had been used since the nineteenth century for diabetes and weight reduction. Theodore Roosevelt used saccharin and fumed when Dr. Wiley told him it was poisonous. Cyclamates were synthesized in 1937 and determined to be thirty times sweeter than sugar. Furthermore, they were chemically stable and inexpensive to produce. Cyclamates had qualified for the GRAS list in 1958, but in 1969, after nearly three decades of safe use, scientists linked the sweetener to cancers found, naturally, in laboratory rats. The FDA promptly invoked the "Delaney Clause," and cyclamates were no longer GRAS. Then in 1977, a Canadian laboratory linked saccharin to bladder cancer in rats; again the

FDA proposed a ban, but diabetics and a weight-conscious electorate pressured legislators. Saccharin remained at the time the
nation's only artificial sweetener.[158]

FDA commissioners subsequent to Dunbar were fully
aware of the problems resulting from enforcement of the Delaney
Clause, but they skirted the issue. In 1972, Commissioner Charles
C. Edwards, a physician with plenty of science education under
his belt, said, "This all or nothing philosophy of the Delaney
Clause sounds reasonable only to the consumer who wants absolute assurance that no harm will come from anything he or she
eats. But we must regulate with the knowledge that absolute safety
is impossible and that science is nearly always incomplete." But
no commissioner until 1996 would hold the power to moderate
Delaney's wording even if he wanted to, and so the clause was rigidly enforced. At the mere mention of circumventing the Delaney
Clause, the agency always heard promptly from Public Citizen
whose *Health Letter* confidently declared, "We need the Delaney
anti-cancer clause . . . humans are 1,000 times more sensitive to
carcinogens than animals." In fact, the evidence proved the oppo-
site was true, but who had time to argue with Sidney Wolfe?[159]

In 1989, the Natural Resources Defense Council delivered
its latest alarmist warning to an audience of fifty million via CBS-
TV's "60 Minutes." Viewers heard Ed Bradley signal that "the
most potent cancer-causing agent in our food supply is a substance sprayed on apples to keep them on trees longer and make
them look better." Daminozide, known commercially as Alar, fed
to mice at 266,000 times normal human consumption of apple
juice, developed benign tumors, placing the spray in violation
of the Delaney Clause. CBS showed footage of children lying in
cancer wards, prompting actress Meryl Streep to lead a crusade
of Mothers and Others for Pesticide Limits. "And so began the
great apple scare," wrote *Washington Times* editorialist Kenneth
Smith, who one year later recalled that the ensuing confiscation
and destruction of apple products had all been for naught except
for costing the apple industry $375 million and American taxpay-
ers $150 million to replace the embargoed apple crop.[160]

The "apple scare," as it would be remembered, contributed to the popularity of a modern food fad, organic farming, largely based on the writings of English agronomist Sir Albert Howard. His 1940 book, *An Agricultural Testament,*" forwards a theory that would have surely earned praise from Harvey Washington Wiley: "Artificial manures lead inevitably to artificial nutrition, artificial food, artificial animals, artificial men and artificial women." Only physical stunting and disease will follow from the expanding use of synthetic fertilizers, he insisted. Given the popular false belief that cancer was epidemic, Howard's ideas were welcomed in America via J. I. Rodale's magazine, *Organic Gardening and Farming* and Wendell Berry's *The Last Whole Earth Catalog.* Within a New Age cultural historical context, a healthy lifestyle depended on knowing where foods were grown and who produced them. "Organic" initially meant locally grown and free of pesticide residues. The organic food movement thumbed its nose at most twentieth-century famine-sparing advances in agronomy and nitrogenous fertilizer development, and would later disparage all efforts to genetically modify seeds despite enormous production advantages and absence of ill effects.

Without a looming public fear of cancer, without a revolution in attitudes about healthful nutrition, without a growing suspicion of the chemical industry, and especially without the Delaney Clause, an obscure laboratory discovery might not have attracted notice from Public Citizen's health vigilante, Sidney Wolfe. During the 1950s when suspected carcinogens were screened by the thousands, two scientists at Columbia University's Institute of Cancer Research saw tumors developing at the site of implanted polymer films. The finding came serendipitously to B. S. and E. T. Oppenheimer, whose experiments were designed to control hypertension. For the first time, a synthetic material considered biologically inert was capable of inducing cancer. Further investigation revealed that other polymers behaved in a similar manner: Ivalon, Dacron, Nylon, Saran, and Teflon. In one of their experiments, implantation of Dow Corning's Silastic elastomer into fifty-four mice yielded fourteen sarcomas. Later called "solid state carcinogenesis," this mode of inducing cancer was documented in scientific journals such as *Science* and *Cancer Research*. Tumor biologists later concluded they were dealing with a mechanical interference of healing generic to most inert materials and not an induction pathway applicable to any clinical cancer. Nonetheless, the biologic identification of an apparent carcinogenic role for the silicone polymers was to have serious clinical, commercial, regulatory, and legal consequences for Dow Corning and other silicone producers. Thanks to the Delaney Amendment, the toxic tort clock was ticking for breast implants.[161]

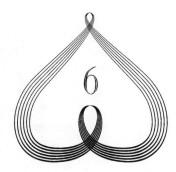

REGULATING THE
MEDICAL DEVICE

*"Man is the only animal that laughs and weeps,
for he is the only animal that knows the difference
between what is and what ought to be."*
—William Hazlitt[162]

When President Roosevelt agreed in 1932 to support legislation expanding the FDA's regulatory dominion, he envisioned a law that would bring cosmetics and medical devices within the agency's jurisdiction. At that time, his advisers were less worried about devices implanted by surgeons than they were suspicious of electronic devices attached to the body for dubious purposes. Fraudulent contraptions had long been foisted upon a gullible public. In eighteenth-century England, John Graham promoted his "celestial bed," whose electrical coils were hyped as a cure for sterility. In 1778, Franz Anton

Mesmer persuaded Parisians to sit for hours in large tubs filled with "magnetized water." But a royal commission that included Antoine Lavoisier and Benjamin Franklin determined that Mesmer was a charlatan. In the United States, the 1872 Postal Fraud Statutes threatened criminal penalties for mail fraud, so the US Postal Service became the only screen for a bogus therapeutic apparatus. Between the two world wars, electronic circuitry became more complex, and the currents required were sufficient to inflict injuries of unprecedented severity. Nonetheless, FDA jurisdiction remained limited to adulteration and misbranding.[163]

During the 1950s, the unanticipated miracles of electronic medical devices included instruments capable of stimulating the rhythmic beat of the human heart. The concept of cardiac pacing was first conceived by Albert Hyman of New York City; in 1932, he built an external hand-operated device for delivery of a carefully timed impulse via needle electrodes passed through the chest wall and attached to the heart muscle. In 1947, Claude Beck first applied a defibrillating current to restore an effective heartbeat, a feat of enormous therapeutic significance. Then in 1958, C. Walton Lillehei at the University of Minnesota successfully treated postoperative heart block with an external pacemaker attached to electrodes placed on the heart's surface. Meanwhile, two Buffalo surgeons, William Chardack and Andrew Gage, worked with engineer Wilson Greatbatch to produce an entirely implantable cardiac pacemaker. Miniaturized with transistor technology, it was powered by mercury-zinc batteries capable of sustaining an effective rhythm for a full year. Because remarkable discoveries like these were appearing concurrently with highly questionable appliances, DHEW Secretary Oveta Culp Hobby appointed a Citizens Advisory Committee to help the FDA examine claims of all device manufacturers. Although electrical inventions attracted the committee's largest concern, silicone devices like the hydrocephalus shunt also came under scrutiny for the first time.[164]

There followed two more mishaps not unlike sulfanilamide—one involving a drug and the other a device—that would garner more power for the FDA, along with adding more layers to the approval process.

Thalidomide was first synthesized in 1953 by a West German firm, Chemie Grunenthal, and marketed as a mild sedative. In liquid format for children, it was considered "West Germany's baby sitter." Thalidomide soon became the most favored sleeping aid, first in Germany and England, then in other European nations and Canada as well. Pregnant women discovered that the drug not only assured sleep but also warded off nausea. Yet, in the United States, both Lederle Laboratories and Smith, Klein, French refused to buy the drug's American license, believing that safety and effectiveness had not been established. Hoffmann-LaRoche also declined because its new tranquilizer, Librium, seemed the better product. A willing licensee was eventually found: William S. Merrell Company of Cincinnati, Ohio, a subsidiary of Vick, hugely famous for its cough drops and VaporRub. Recognizing the success of thalidomide in foreign markets, Merrell's medical director, Joseph Murray (not the Nobelist Joseph Murray) looked forward to a lucrative American market and asked for an expedited review.[165]

After filing his new drug application (NDA) on September 12, 1960, Murray met with immediate resistance from Dr. Frances O. Kelsey, newly appointed as a drug reviewer. Although a medical graduate, and before that earning a doctorate in pharmacology, she lacked job experience and needed help; it was her first encounter with an entirely new drug. The 1938 law stipulated that an application would receive automatic approval sixty days following submission unless it was found scientifically lacking, in which case it could be withdrawn and resubmitted. Believing that the studies supporting the application were more like testimonials than scientific evidence, she declared the NDA inadequate two days short of the deadline. Time and again she used the sixty-day rule to keep the drug off the market. Clearly, she was learning about regulatory procedure; this remains a recognized FDA delay tactic in use today.

Chemie Grunenthal withdrew thalidomide from the German market on November 20, 1961, fourteen months after the initial NDA filing, following reports of severe congenital malformations. When informed, Kelsey elected to wait for more evidence. In fact, no one at the agency responded as the FDA had done in 1938 following the sulfanilamide tragedy. Instead, a winter passed without further action. On February 21, 1962, the president of the Merrell Company wrote to physicians in Canada where the drug remained available: "There is still no positive proof of a causal relationship between the use of thalidomide during pregnancy and malformations in the newborn." At the time of his letter, there were two thousand malformed babies born of mothers using thalidomide in Europe.[166]

In April 1962, Dr. Helen Taussig, a distinguished professor of pediatrics at Johns Hopkins University, contacted Dr. John Nestor at the FDA with a personal account of long bone deformities witnessed during her recent European journey. Nestor forwarded the information to Kelsey, who wrote to Murray asking how many American doctors were enrolled in thalidomide trials. Expecting at most thirty, she learned that more than a thousand had been given tablets for use by their patients. Yet, she still did not act on the information. After Dr. Taussig reported her findings to the American College of Physicians, the story was picked up by the press and congressional action was soon under way. Not until July 23, 1962, eight months after Merrell informed the FDA that the drug had been withdrawn from the German market, did Commissioner George P. Larrick send inspectors to Cincinnati, where they uncovered deceptions that would shock Congress, the American public, and the legitimate pharmaceutical industry.[167]

Merrell's marketing department, not its medical department, had organized the clinical research in a manner that produced the most expansive clinical trial in history with 1,267 physicians enrolled, not all of them prepared to provide accurate lists of their patients. An estimated twenty thousand had already consumed 2.5 million tablets. Merrell suffered a landslide of civil litigation unprecedented in American pharmaceutical history. Company executives acknowledged that five tons had been imported but only three tons accounted for. The FDA turned to the American Medical Association (AMA) for help notifying physicians of the danger.[168]

A comprehensive report appeared on the front page of the *Washington Post* assigning full credit to Dr. Kelsey for averting disaster: "Heroine of the FDA Keeps Bad Drug Off Market." The story spread rapidly throughout the mass media. At a press conference, President John F. Kennedy urged women everywhere to search for and dispose of any strange drugs in their medicine chests. In the United States alone, more than six hundred women became pregnant after receiving the drug, but only seventeen cases of phocomelia were documented, seven resulting from the use of drug purchased outside the country. In Germany, the toll was thirty-five hundred deformed babies, an outbreak so large and sudden that hereditary factors could be ruled out. Before the thalidomide tragedy reached closure, Commissioner Larrick was permitted to retire quietly, while Dr. Kelsey received a Distinguished Federal Service Gold Medal.[169]

The horror of thalidomide is still remembered as a debacle for the drug industry and a singular victory for government regulation. Few recall that no less than three major pharmaceutical firms had seen inadequate testing by Chemie Grunenthal and refused to bid for the drug's American license. In the final analysis, the FDA's role was limited to passive resistance. Like elixir sulfanilamide, thalidomide served to galvanize congressional attention to further amend the law. Missing from the 1938 act was unconditional authority to withhold approval of a drug, indefinitely if necessary, until proof of safety was firmly established. The 1962 amendments converted the regulation of drugs from premarket notification to premarket approval, an important legal distinction. No longer would marketing and distribution proceed automatically after a sixty-day waiting period. Moreover, proof of efficacy became a requirement; new drugs had to be compliant with every therapeutic benefit claimed by the manufacturer.

Meanwhile, a companion bill that required similar provisions for all medical devices was withdrawn at the last moment, but with agreement that Congress should return to the matter of device legislation within a few months. Another fifteen years passed before that step was taken. President Lyndon B. Johnson urged new medical device authority in a consumer safety message. When Richard M. Nixon later omitted reference to the need for a stronger device law, a Democratic Party task force forced him to do so. After congressional testimony in 1969 revealed x-ray machines without proper radiation safeguards, Nixon became his own advocate for stronger device oversight.[170]

Later that year, the Supreme Court unwittingly accelerated device regulation by issuing a decision that confounded prior distinctions between drugs and devices. In *United States v. Bacto Unidisk*, tiny discs used for laboratory determination of antibiotic sensitivity were declared a drug, not a device, according to the precedent of surgical sutures being regulated as drugs. But it was a judicial position that would not prevail for long. A concurrent DHEW study group chaired by National Heart Institute Director Theodore Cooper concluded that medical devices were a different kind of regulatory challenge and deserved independent statutory language. The Cooper Committee urged an immediate inventory of all medical devices in current use, and a systematic categorization that distinguished products requiring premarket approval from all others safely held to general performance standards. Implicit in their proposal was an expectation that some devices already in the marketplace would be designated for review as if they were brand new. This was the boldest move yet proposed for regulation of medical devices because it meant that industries would be faced with securing retroactive approval for a portion of their existing product line. During the debate that followed this proposal, advocates for the stronger law were granted a timely gift: the Dalkon Shield affair, yet another tragedy leading to more regulatory power.[171]

Intrauterine contraceptive devices (IUDs) were not new to the 1970s; millions had already been implanted in the form of coils, bows, rings, spirals, loops, and springs. In 1968, Dr. Hugh J. Davis, director of the Family Planning Clinic at Johns Hopkins Hospital, established a business association with an electrical engineer, Irwin Lerner, and an attorney, Robert Cohn. Lerner had recently patented a variation of the doctor's own successful invention, the "Incon Ring" device. Dr. Davis thus became a silent business partner in the Dalkon Corporation ('Da' for Davis, 'L' for Lerner, and 'Kon' for Cohn). The company's only product was the Dalkon Shield, an IUD that added a membrane and spikes to the original framework. Because the new patent was in Lerner's name alone, Davis stopped sharing profits with Johns Hopkins as he was still required to do.[172]

Now his university clinic suddenly transferred its allegiance from the Incon Ring to the Dalkon Shield. Comparing his experience with both devices, Davis reported in the *American Journal of Obstetrics and Gynecology* that side effects were minimal and conception rate much lower (1.1 percent) for the Dalkon Shield. Another journal mistakenly reported a 0.5 percent pregnancy rate, lower than any prior experience. Davis not only failed to correct that error but later admitted the rate was actually 6 percent. Yet he continued to use the 1.1 percent rate for marketing purposes. Meanwhile, the FDA was receiving reports of severe pelvic infections, uterine perforations, septicemia, and deaths following use of IUDs. Because no correlation existed between complications and any specific device on the market, no warnings were issued at the time.

In the wake of Commissioner Larrick's resignation and the election of Richard M. Nixon, a corporate style search for new leadership was conducted. Charles C. Edwards, the first physician ever considered for the job, enjoyed prior government experience (CIA) and had served as a staff surgeon at the Mayo Clinic. After a term as director of programs for the AMA, he joined the business consultant firm Booz-Allen and Hamilton. Following confirmation, Edwards turned to the private sector for legal counsel and found Peter Barton Hutt, a highly regarded advocate for industry in regulatory matters and a partner at Covington Burling in Washington, DC. Democrats in Congress were understandably concerned that wolves were assuming responsibility for guarding the hen house. In fact, the commissioner's team embraced its responsibilities fully, and instituted the kind of management principles the FDA had not previously experienced. Edwards was a man who preferred direct and frequent contact with the industries his agency was dealing with. He found the FDA both understaffed and underbudgeted for its responsibilities; only fourteen medical officers were responsible for reviewing twenty-five hundred applications each year. Given his prior experience and a facility for dealing with legislators, Edwards achieved what was believed impossible: a doubling of the FDA budget inside of two years.[173]

Meanwhile, Hutt addressed persisting legal issues, among them data confidentiality. An emerging consumer movement and passage of the Freedom of Information Act produced countless demands from advocacy groups for information about drug effectiveness. Hutt established new rules limiting confidentiality to recently submitted applications, thus opening 90 percent of the FDA's information base to the public. This development alone prompted an avalanche of inquires, forty-five thousand in the first year, costing the agency over one million dollars.

Unlike most of his predecessors, Commissioner Edwards met almost daily with senior staff to define objectives and survey progress. He recruited dozens of new professionals, modernized outdated laboratories, and built on the established principle of external advisory panels. Anticipating passage of stronger medical device legislation, he recruited panels for classifying all devices in current use. The Advisory Committee Act of 1972 established guidelines for selecting qualified experts, and the Sunshine in Government Act assured that government hearings were open to the public. By 1974, there were sixty-six functioning advisory committees, each meeting for two days at least twice yearly. Among them were the General and Plastic Surgery Devices Advisory Panel whose job was to survey every device in modern surgical practice, from bandages to operating room kick buckets, cardiac pacemakers and, in time, breast implants. At the same time, the Obstetrics and Gynecology Advisory Panel was kept busy with an avalanche of complaints from patients with IUDs.[174]

In 1970, Dr. Davis and his business partners attracted commercial interest in their shield from A. H. Robins in Richmond,

Virginia. Despite discrepancies in pregnancy rates, executives remained keen on purchasing the Dalkon Corporation. The three partners were assigned a 10 percent stake in the profits, a fact that Davis would later deny in testimony before Congress. Next, Robins' engineers altered the configuration of the Dalkon Shield, thinning the membrane, rounding the spikes, and strengthening the multifilamentous structure with copper, a known adjunct to contraception. Without any effectiveness data for the modified device, they began selling the product immediately.

The FDA was still accumulating reports of pelvic inflammation and uterine perforations. Faced with explaining to the House Intergovernmental Relations Committee how it was dealing with the IUD problem, the FDA resorted to product seizure, a tactic that had always worked for the agency in the past. On May 25, 1975, US marshals seized nine thousand uterine devices from a Jamaica, New York, warehouse. Meanwhile, the FDA was awaiting passage of a Medical Device Amendments, one that was faithful to the principles of the Cooper Committee. Peter Hutt insisted that the process must begin with a systematic classification of all the devices in use. Furthermore, there must be a provision for selective scrutiny of problem devices already in use, as the damage caused by the Dalkon Shield had recently confirmed. When the bill was passed by the Senate in April 1975 and the House in March 1976, its final language was remarkably faithful to the Cooper Committee recommendations. There would be a review and classification of every device in use, some of them subject to further scrutiny. When President Gerald Ford signed the amendment into law on May 28, 1976, A. H. Robins already faced more than six hundred lawsuits. Anticipating an agency empowered by the new device amendments, the company discontinued manufacture of the Dalkon Shield for its American market, but it continued to sell its existing inventory to foreign nations. Not until 1980, ten years after purchasing the Dalkon Corporation, did Robins officials advise removal of the devices.[175]

Resistance to stronger regulatory laws can be thought of as a natural corporate reflex. In a democratic society, enterprising executives become accustomed to having their own way. Just as Coca-Cola's Asa Candler could not tolerate a government agency telling him how to run his business, H. J. Heinz couldn't imagine any regulator knowing more about ketchup than he did. On the other hand, George Merck had no difficulty meeting the standards imposed by the 1938 act (although he later felt the burden of costs associated with delayed approvals). Only when a corporation dominates a market can it safely support higher regulation standards, thereby reducing competition. There is no evidence that Dow Corning lobbied against the device amendments. In fact, management believed there was little to fear from a regulatory agency.[176]

General Electric, on the other hand, reacted differently to the Medical Device Amendments. Their Waterford, New York, plant was second to Dow Corning for silicone production capacity. Smaller medical product manufacturers who competed with Dow Corning preferred to buy their unprocessed polymer from GE, which led executives in Waterford to consider investing the necessary capital to upgrade their plant and broaden their product line. Discussing the prospect with Jack Welch, vice president for chemicals and plastics soon to be appointed CEO, General Manager for Silicone Products Tom Fitzgerald outlined the anticipated regulatory and liability burdens and argued for GE to remove itself from the medical device field in favor of expanding production capacity in their established markets. It was a historic decision that Welch and fellow executives later congratulated themselves for making.[177]

GE's revised strategy did not mean that Dow Corning could enjoy its dominant position in the medical sector without fighting to sustain it. Competition loomed in the form of smaller companies focused exclusively on medical devices. They included Heyer-Schulte, McGhan Medical, and Cox-Uphoff, all based in Santa Barbara, California; Medical Engineering Corporation in Racine, Wisconsin, Mentor Corporation in Minneapolis, Minnesota, and the French-owned company, Simaplast. Each competitor based its strategic planning on continued innovation using former Dow Corning chemists and engineers. The advantages of working in a young organization instead of a large corporation appealed to inventive people like Don McGhan and Dick Compton, Jim Cox and Bob Uphoff, all representing the "young Turks" in a burgeoning industrial sector.

When the device amendments became law, the General and Plastic Surgery Devices Panel had been meeting in Washington for nearly two years under the chairmanship of J. B. Lynch, chairman of the Department of Plastic Surgery at Vanderbilt University. Its members included practicing surgeons as well as experts in fields such as biomaterials science, pathology, microbiology, and oncology. A research scientist from Johnson & Johnson served as the industry representative. Consumer advocates attended meetings, as did an FDA staff member. Dow Corning sent Arthur Rathjen to monitor the proceedings. Following the agenda of the Cooper Committee, the committee listed every surgical device and categorized them according to these definitions:

Class I: Devices used external to the body, such as surgical instruments and wound dressings that require limited controls.

Class II: Devices such as sutures, with a function that require performance standards.

Class III: Devices with a potential for hazard, including all that are intended for surgical implantation. New products always required premarket approval (PMA), and some were destined for PMA despite their long record in the marketplace.[178]

Advisory panels could easily comply with the required inventories but didn't always agree with the proposed class designations. The General and Plastic Devices Panel agreed with Class III for cardiac pacemakers but held that Class II was more appropriate for the breast implant given its longstanding use and a low complication rate. Dow Corning's management welcomed the participation of medical professionals in the classification dialogue. The enormous costs of submitting a PMA guaranteed the cooperation of the smaller producers as well. A close working relationship between industry and the American Society of Plastic and Reconstructive Surgeons (ASPRS) followed. Few surgeons at the time questioned whether by avoiding a premarket review, they were acting on behalf of their patients or in support of industry. A day would come, however, when most ASPRS members wished they could shed their corporate partnership image.[179]

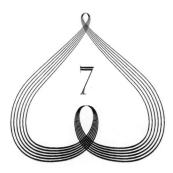

BALANCING
CLINICAL RISK WITH
CLINICAL BENEFIT

"Primum non nocere!"
—Hippocrates[180]

"We are all prisoners of life under sentence of death."
—J. B. S. Haldane[181]

Hippocrates' immortal caveat, "First, do no harm," was imparted at a time when the physician's role in society was a privileged one, and individual rights were subordinated to a central authority. On matters of health, patients in the time of Hippocrates did not engage in the decision-making process; they didn't even enjoy the privilege of learning what little was known about their illness. Informed consent was not feasible because risk wasn't considered measurable or manageable. Risks happened at the whim of the gods; the future was the domain of oracles and soothsayers. In time there came a revolutionary change, leading to a compulsive need to control risk. Modern man is no longer passive before nature but strives to understand risk and weigh its consequences.[182]

Implicit in the oath that has come down to us from Hippocrates is an exclusive one-on-one relationship that, regrettably, bears no resemblance to the contemporary medical model. Nowadays the patient's personal physician may not even be the most appropriate specialist to administer optimum treatment. Effective treatment of the infirm or the injured now involves a collaborative network of health professionals, each one qualified to impart some but not all of the knowledge a patient is entitled by law to be told. Every member of the team contributes to a collective understanding of risk, now referred to as informed consent. But information pertaining to sickness and health, in the past dispensed only by physicians, is now available to patients from many sources, none of them imagined in the days of Hippocrates: newspapers and other popular publications, each filtered by an editor faced with limited space; books whose content is the product of writers often unqualified for the task; television news reports limited to ninety seconds at most, with a premium awarded for sensationalism; and an expanding World Wide Web filled with unconfirmed assertions. Not one of these can fully substitute for the carefully measured advice of an informed and caring physician or nurse practitioner. In order to understand and manage risk, today's patient must accept that modern medical therapy is always prone to unwitting error and unavoidable risk. Furthermore, the vagaries of human nature provide ample opportunity for witting error and avoidable risk. Nonetheless, the relevance of the great physician's oath endures, and the admonition it conveys to modern healers is clear: make every effort to avoid bringing harm to your patient.

The catch, however, is this: harm is a subjective measure and risk is relative. Some individuals are remarkably risk tolerant, while others are intensely risk adverse. Moreover, ours is a society capable of either overreacting to imagined risk or overlooking genuine risk. Beef consumption can take a nosedive following the solitary occurrence of "mad-cow disease," while thousands suffer E. coli enteritis each year because of enduring flaws in the Meat Inspection Act of 1906. Unimagined catastrophes like those of September 11, 2001, that took the lives of 265 commercial jet occupants can bring the airline industry to the brink of financial ruin, while an even larger motor vehicle death toll recorded after any weekend in America barely elicits special concern except from those dear to the victims. Trace quantities of pesticides in the food supply without documented health risk serve to guarantee the formidable success of today's organic food retailers, while the increased risk of type 2 diabetes or death from coronary heart disease arouses minimum interest in making lifestyle changes known to reduce cardiovascular diseases. These are not recent behavioral trends. In the early days of food and drug oversight, Harvey Washington Wiley's inspectors focused their efforts on unproven risks such as "fraudulent" sugar, blended whiskey, and excess caffeine in soft drinks. Meanwhile, the risk of death from contagion was omnipresent, and vaccination programs were poorly administered. Today, mortality resulting from contagion is rare but growing once again in America. Why? Because effective immunization programs are challenged by an erroneous fear that childhood autism is caused by modern vaccines. Public reaction to risk is based on stories rather than facts and fails to correlate with the reality of risk, which is not often enough expressed as relative risk.[183]

Physicians have traditionally based their art on an imperfectly defined balance between relative benefit and relative risk. Meanwhile, important external influences come into play: the profit motive favors benefits and minimizes risk while anticorporate bias minimizes benefit and exaggerates risks. Not only physicians, scientists and other innovators but also journalists, legislators, and eventually regulators all contribute to deliberations influencing both sides of the risk equation. In time, attorneys and insurance underwriters add their own interests, prejudices, and costs to an already complex interaction. The management of risk in both liberal and totalitarian societies inevitably becomes far more political than scientific in character.

The modern conception of risk and its rational management is rooted in a Hindu-Arabic numbering system that allowed for the first serious mathematical consideration of risk during the Renaissance. The discovery of probability theory by Blaise Pascal and Pierre de Fermat encouraged reliable forecasting of future events, essential for effective commercial trade. Examples include the estimation of future crop yields and the likelihood of ships returning safely. Marine insurance soon followed. Jacob Bernouli's "law of large numbers" led to statistical sampling, and Abraham Moivre gave the world the normal distribution of data (a.k.a. the bell curve), as well as the concept of standardized deviation. Then, Francis Galton contributed "regression to the mean," which allows for decision making based on the likelihood of certain events returning to an average frequency. From these important working theorems have come the calculation of life tables, insurance underwriting, diversified investing, business projecting, and game theories of endless variety. In the final analysis, however, it is an individual's inherent feeling of comfort or mounting fear that determines their personal estimation of risk.[184]

Dr. Cronin did not mention risk potential in his written report published in the proceedings of the Washington Congress of Plastic Surgeons. In fact, he did not even list how many patients had already been implanted, believing that his was an expanding clinical experience he would keep track of and document in follow-up reports. Meanwhile, Dow Corning incorporated Cronin's updates into their product information document (PID) and assumed plastic surgeons were passing it on for their patients' understanding. Most of them were. By the late 1960s, informed consent was fully adopted for medical risk management.[185]

Early PIDs listed three categories of risk for patients seeking breast enlargement. First, there were the problems associated with any surgical procedure: pain, bleeding, postoperative infection, and the inevitability of a permanent surgical scar. A second category included risks following use of any medical device, principally an increased risk of infection associated with implanting a foreign material. Third, there were the risks specific to a silicone breast implant: dissatisfaction, asymmetry, and diminished nipple sensation, most of these uncommon or temporary. More frequent was a fibrotic reaction not unlike those following use of the porous plastic devices but limited to the surface of the implant where a fibrous capsule always formed. Patients started out with a soft breast that might later become firmer, but not as hardened as with the sponge devices. Not everyone developed firmer breasts, but "capsular contraction" soon became a primary concern for patients wanting implants, surgeons willing to put them in, and manufacturers striving for a flawless product.[186]

Dr. Cronin always reminded his younger colleagues that postoperative problems had been more troublesome when he used the Ivalon sponge device; silicone gel was far superior. After all, there was no absorption of body fluid. And regardless of the outcome, patient satisfaction was primarily linked to their new body profile. He enjoyed paraphrasing one delighted patient, an exotic dancer: "For every one who feels them, there are hundreds who sees them."[187]

The task of examining patients implanted with the Cronin device and tabulating their outcomes was assigned to one of his residents, Roger Greenberg. Of 183 patients with a mean age of thirty years, nearly every one was married at the time of surgery. Their motivation was usually underdevelopment of one or both breasts or else loss of shape and volume following pregnancy. Most women asked for an appropriate body proportion rather than exceptionally large breasts. Most patients were implanted in sizes ranging from 220 cc (7 ounces) to 260 cc (9 ounces). The smallest device used was 120 cc and the largest 450 cc. There were two episodes of postoperative bleeding and seven postoperative infections requiring implant removal with subsequent reimplantation. Less common were mechanical problems, such as a poorly positioned implant and in one case, wound separation with exposure requiring device removal. Overall, 85 percent of patients were classified good to excellent meaning soft and well-positioned breasts without complications. Fifteen percent were classed as fair to poor, meaning firm breasts or else a positioning error or post-operative complication. Despite the problem, patient acceptance was unanimous; nobody asked for removal.[188]

Meanwhile, demand for breast enlargement surgery continued to grow throughout the 1970s. Because medical advertising was still believed unethical, the popularity of breast implants depended entirely on word-of-mouth testimonials. Breast implant scuttlebutt passed quickly from grateful patients to curious friends. Clinical results, by all popular accounts, were superb. Women previously shy about telling anyone about their breast surgery were more willing to discuss their experience with others; some even displayed their new breasts to close friends. While its popularity grew, the device itself continued to improve. Palpable seams were eliminated and the protective shell became thinner but stronger. Also, the gel was becoming more responsive to touch and therefore a closer approximation of natural breast tissue.

But at the same time breast firmness following surgery remained the most common source of patient disappointment, occasionally requiring reoperation. Because intense fibrous reactions were sometimes observed near the Dacron fixation patches, Gerow asked Dow Corning engineers to remove them. They weren't needed for maintaining implant position. Although most patients delighted in their new breast profiles and believed any firmness was more a side effect than a complication, plastic surgeons and manufacturers set their minds to eliminating the issue.

The continuing quest for reliably softer implanted breasts notwithstanding, the stunning success of silicone polymers for breast enlargement surgery attracted other device innovators. In 1969, Roger Klein brought to the American market a saline inflatable device manufactured by Simaplast of France. Named for its inventive surgeon, the Arion device was little more than a silicone shell with a filling catheter that gave surgeons intra-operative flexibility. Once the desired volume was reached, the catheter was removed at its base and the aperture sealed. One disadvantage of the device was valve failure, deflation, and a need for implant replacement. At about this time, Heyer-Schulte

Corporation recruited Don McGhan, a mechanical engineer from Dow Corning, who with plastic surgery collaboration, produced a seamless inflatable device with a more reliable valve and fewer deflations than previous designs.[189]

Among the advantages claimed for saline-filled devices was a softer breast. Capsule contraction was thus linked to use of silicone gel, leading to speculation that subtle leakage of polymer droplets into the surrounding tissue explained the fibrous reaction. Dow Corning's so-called dielectric gel was of hybrid composition: short chains held within a matrix of longer chains. At the surface of the gel, some shorter chain molecules could break free and pass through the outer shell. This was the leeching that Dr. Cronin had been cautioned about. Eventually the term "gel bleed," was applied to this phenomenon.[190]

The marketplace, although still dominated by Dow Corning, saw entry of more manufacturers offering a variety of competing products: gel vs. saline, round vs. teardrop, thick shell vs. thin. As surgeons acquired experience with different devices, claims of superiority became ardent and contradictory. In the midst of this confusion, Florida plastic surgeon James Baker conducted a patient study not since duplicated. Acknowledging the importance of controlled experiments, he offered eligible women an augmentation mammaplasty without a surgical fee if they would allow him to place dissimilar implants behind each breast. Fifty-nine volunteered, and a software program guaranteed random pairings: different manufacturers, different shapes, etc. Although he promised a replacement without charge for any unacceptable symmetry, all but one were content with their first set of implants. Baker had confirmed Cronin's observation that it was improved contour that determined satisfaction. Another lesson was that breast implants, despite their featured production differences, were less noticeably variable behind normal breast tissue.[191]

Surgeons sometimes misused their own terminology, such as when capsule, contraction, and contracture were applied interchangeably. The semantic distinction is important. The capsule or membrane forms around every implanted device. Contraction refers to modest firmness; contracture indicates more severe contraction. Dr. Baker defined four degrees of capsule pathology:

> Class I—"Breast absolutely natural; cannot tell breast
>   is surgically augmented"
> Class II—"Minimal contraction; can tell surgery was
>   performed, but without complaint"
> Class III—"Moderate contraction; patient definitely
>   feels some firmness"
> Class IV—"Severe contracture with breast distortion"

In so doing, he transformed postoperative complication reporting. The Baker I–IV Classification remains the accepted standard for grading the outcome of breast implantation.[192]

Ross Rudolph, a plastic surgeon at the University of California–San Diego (UCSD), was interested in biologic mechanisms of wound contraction, a phenomenon well known to influence the quality of skin graft healing in burn victims. Microscopic examination of healing grafts revealed myofibroblasts, specialized cells with contractile properties similar to those of muscle cells. After finding these cells in capsules encircling heart pacemakers, Rudolph looked for and found the same cells in the membranes surrounding breast implants. Perhaps their presence explained the mechanism of contraction. Aware of the theory that gel bleed caused capsule formation, he collected membrane biopsies and asked pathologist Jerrold Abraham to look for silicone. Abraham used x-rays to confirm that the capsules held elemental silicon. With no other reason to find silicon in human scar tissue, Rudolph concluded that it was silicone that leaked into the capsules. Calculations revealed that only a few grams of silicone (a minute fraction of an ounce) were present. When a chemical equilibrium was reached, silicone no longer migrated into the capsule, indicating that gel bleed was not a continuous phenomenon. More important, Dr. Rudolph found no correlation between capsular silicone and breast firmness. Some patients with silicone in their capsules maintained soft breasts while others showing negligible

| *Before* | *After* |

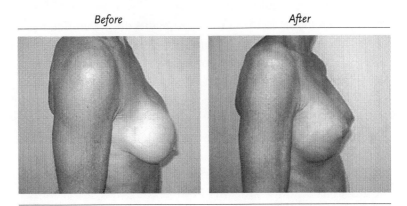

After multiple pregnancies and earlier breast implants, a 56 yr. old grand-mother is unhappy with her firm, spherical, drooping breasts. Baker Class IV contracted capsules released, ptosis corrected with bilateral mastopexy, and implants replaced. CREDIT: Anne Wallace MD

leakage experienced firm breasts. What this meant was that sili-cone in capsules was incidental to contraction and not its cause.[193]

Tucson, Arizona, plastic surgeon, Boyd Burkhardt posit-ed in an editorial that clinically detectable contraction following mammary augmentation was a breast-specific rather than a patient-specific phenomenon. He based this on the observation that capsule contraction sometimes developed in one breast but not in the other. Burkhardt theorized that factors other than a patient's overall sensitivity to a foreign implant were at work. He stood among a small but growing number of surgeons who pre-ferred saline inflatable implants. Patients informed of leakage potential were sometimes repelled by the idea and asked for the saline option. Heyer Schulte's Don McGhan collaborated with silicone chemist Dick Compton to establish NuSil, a new man-ufacturer of silicone polymers, and patented a phenyl-silicone version of the elastomer shell with one-tenth prior levels of mem-brane permeability. Yet, contraction remained a problem despite these innovations; no surprise to Dr. Rudolph. His conclusion that gel bleed had little to do with contraction was not yet widely accepted.[194]

In the midst of concerns about gel bleed, reports of breast cancers developing in women with implants drew attention to silicone's uncommon role as a carcinogen. Pleas for surgeon restraint in the face of a possible cancer risk were not new; they were voiced back in the days of porous plastic implants: "Operations on Bosoms Dangerous," declared Dr. Walter Alvarez in a 1954 *Los Angeles Times* feature. A noted health authority, Alvarez was supported by California plastic surgeon W. W. Kiskadden. But theoretical objections of this kind were easily ignored in a city where physical appearance was paramount. Then in 1967, plastic surgeons at Johns Hopkins Hospital reported on six women implanted with both Ivalon and silicone implants who developed breast cancer. The authors stopped short of attributing the cancers to any single synthetic exposure. But they did issue a warning that implants might impede cancer detection.[195]

Intense warnings came later from Dr. June Marchant of the British Cancer Registry. In a letter published in the July 26, 1975, issue of *Lancet,* she cited the experimental work of the Oppenheimers with solid state carcinogenesis. She urged caution when considering the use of any foreign material in proximity to breast tissue. Omitted from her analysis was acknowledgement that solid state carcinogens had induced only fibrous sarcomas and never breast cancer.[196]

Additional case reports of cancer developing in women with implants led to a remarkable collaboration between Los Angeles plastic surgeon Garry Brody and the University of Southern California (USC) School of Public Health. During a chance encounter with USC epidemiologist Bruce Henderson in 1974, Brody asked whether a study could be designed to determine whether breast cancer risk was influenced by silicone exposure. Henderson, who had recently established a cancer registry for Los Angeles County, referred Brody to fellow epidemiologist Malcolm Pike, who explained two methods: the case-control study and the cohort study. There were advantages and disadvantages to each.

The term "case-control study" did not appear in the medical literature until 1967; yet precedents for the method were established in the nineteenth century with the advent of defining human illness according to common diagnostic criteria. Thomas Sydenham, sometimes referred to as the British Hippocrates, was a forceful advocate of distinguishing diseases according to their symptoms, signs, and clinical course. This unitary concept of illness contrasted sharply with antiquarian beliefs that "fever," for example, was itself a uniform malady that never varied. An organized study of a single disease process as it affected one or more victims required first, an accurate medical history, which in turn allowed for comparisons between individuals or groups. In 1855, Dr. John Snow asked families of cholera victims about the habits of decedents and determined that risk of contracting the disease and dying from its effects was closely related to the drawing of water from a particular town pump. In the twentieth century, the modern case-control format was established by Janet Lane-Claypon, whose British Medical Research Council study determined that diminished fertility increased the risk of breast cancer.[197]

In contrast to the retrospective case-control strategy, the cohort study model is more often prospective because subjects are characterized prior to the onset of disease and then followed for as many years as needed. Cohort studies hold the advantage of eliminating sources of bias that can influence case-control analysis. The principal disadvantage is that large populations must be followed for many years to achieve valid results.[198]

Based on Professor Pike's advice, Dr. Brody's best strategy was clear. Silicone breast implantation was the exposure in question, and breast cancer was the suspected outcome. This required a prospective cohort design, meaning that thousands of women with silicone mammary devices were needed, all of them tracked for several years. It seemed a daunting task, given that privacy issues always accompany breast surgery. Brody began by soliciting the participation of plastic surgeons throughout Los Angeles County, especially those with large private cosmetic practices. Nearly fifty expressed interest but with the proviso that patient confidentiality be maintained. Women pursuing breast enlargement surgery often want no one but their plastic surgeon and perhaps a family member to know anything about their surgery. Some patients actually withhold knowledge of prior breast surgery from spouses present and future. Mailing a health questionnaire was out of the question. To reveal a patient's name without permission would represent a violation of trust.[199]

Fortunately, the public health code of the State of California provided a mechanism for collecting health facts without revealing other details about the patient's personal medical history. This statute had long served the public as a means of studying patterns of communicable diseases. The Los Angeles County Cancer Surveillance Program (CSP), established by Bruce Henderson, was entirely dependent on the same code mandating the reporting of all new cancer diagnoses by every licensed physician in the county. Dr. Pike offered Dr. Brody the assistance of Dennis Deapen, a doctoral candidate in epidemiology, who agreed to conduct the implant cancer risk study. As a sworn public health officer, only Deapen was permitted access to the names of patients who had received breast implants, along with their age and the date of surgery. For assurance of confidentiality, the law stipulated that patients could not be contacted or even informed that they were part of a research investigation. This meant that potential cofactors such as family history, age at menarche, and history of pregnancy would not be available to the investigators for analysis. A subject's name could be used by Deapen but only for the purpose of computer matching with the CSP roster of registered breast cancer patients. After a period of years, this information would permit a comparison of expected risk, with the actual cancer risk observed among implant recipients. Continued enrollment in the study also required confirmation of local residence, obtained either from voter registration rolls, property tax rolls, or the Department of Motor Vehicles.

Professor Pike was invited to explain the privacy safeguards at a meeting of the California Plastic Surgery Society. Largely because of his reassurances, thirty-five plastic surgeons remained enrolled in the project. Initial funding came from USC and from Dr. Brody himself. How many years of follow-up would be required? It all depended on how many subjects stayed enrolled; participating surgeons hoped they might be able to assemble the names of ten thousand implant recipients over the span of a decade. Data collection began late in 1974.[200]

In the meantime, what were women who expressed interest in breast enlargement being told about the risks of silicone implants? The 1970s, a decade that produced a far better understanding of breast implant outcomes, were also years when medical malpractice litigation reached crisis levels and a corporation's legal obligation to warn users about the risks of their products became universal. But confidentiality standards prevented manufacturers from knowing the names of patients who received their products. Therefore, a corporation's duty to warn was fulfilled by informing the implanting surgeon. And so the document originally composed by Dr. Cronin for the benefit of surgeons using the first implants gradually evolved into the manufacturer's product information document (PID), commonly referred to as the "package insert." Its content included basic facts about chemical composition, physical specifications, instructions for use, contraindications, precautions, and known complications.

Early in the 1970s, PIDs were long on specifications but lean on risk experience; manufacturers were dependent on plastic surgeons for documenting complications. Other than Dr. Cronin's follow-up reporting, outcome data for breast implant surgery remained scarce. Individual case reports were plentiful, but accounts of consecutive patient experiences were lacking. As this information was reported and published, the scope of the package inserts expanded. Although rupture was listed as a risk, these were still uncommon events. Deflation of saline-filled implants was common enough to justify mention in every package insert. Nothing about leakage of silicone was initially mentioned (the term "gel bleed" wasn't used prior to 1975). Throughout the 1980s, corporate attorneys began to recommend listing every incident ever reported, whether related to the implant or not, thus stripping the insert of its information effectiveness. The duty to warn had become a ritual for protecting the enterprise instead of a vehicle for informing the surgeon or the patient.[201]

Plastic surgeons were sometimes responsible for aggravating a manufacturer's concerns about device safety. James Baker related an incident involving one of his breast augmentation patients, a former Miss Colorado, who received an impromptu bear hug from an admirer, felt a sudden pop in her breasts, and later noticed her firm breasts were soft again. Baker's published description led to widespread adoption of an office procedure called manual capsulotomy: deliberate compression of a firm breast to release the capsule, expand the space available for the implant, and produce the desired outcome, a softer breast. The risks for this procedure, although rare, included bleeding and even damage to the implant itself. Manufacturers refused to accept this risk and began warning against its use in their package insert.[202]

When Thomas Biggs became Dr. Cronin's partner, he assumed responsibility for tabulating the group's combined experience with the device. Reporting in 1980 an eighteen-year experience with 1,567 patients, 98 percent reported satisfaction without need for reoperation despite many who experienced breast firmness. Placing calls to those who failed to respond, Biggs found a few more patients who were not pleased with their surgery, more often because their motive for implants had been to satisfy someone else's need, not their own.[203]

One of the patients he interviewed was their first patient, Timmie Jean Lindsay. "It wasn't anything I couldn't live without," she told Dr. Biggs. But she fondly recalled wolf whistles on the street soon after. Mrs. Lindsay expressed full satisfaction with her surgery at a time when others claimed health problems. "I was a guinea pig, but I was treated so royally I didn't feel like one." For Mrs. Lindsay, the good that came from her decision justified any risk she had taken.[204]

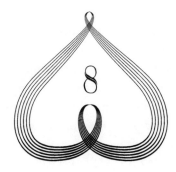

DOW CORNING
UNDER SIEGE

*"It is not our policy to inform the FDA of anything
we are not required by law to tell them."*
—Robert Rylee, Dow Corning, 1989[205]

When the Medical Device Amendments became law in 1976, Midland's second corporate giant (after Dow Chemical) was entering its fourth decade of continuous innovation and prosperity, even in the face of an economic recession. Although the company was forced to compete aggressively with other manufacturers of silicones for industrial applications, it dominated the medical products field. Ever since its wartime role as a pioneer in polymer chemistry, Dow Corning enjoyed the self-confidence of an enterprise whose contributions to aerospace, advanced electronics, and state-of-the-art medical care had never been challenged. Nonetheless, Dow Corning was a corporate innocent in the face of advancing regulatory power, unrestrained consumer activism, and mass tort litigation.

Led by visionary executives with unquestioned scientific pedigrees, Dow Corning's annual revenue had grown from forty million dollars in 1950 to seven hundred million dollars by 1980. Yet, medical products represented less than 5 percent of sales, and breast implants would never yield more than 1 percent of the company's income. Dow Corning's employees were a conspicuously proud assembly of managers, chemists, and engineers, supported by a highly specialized staff uniformly aware of Dow Corning's pathfinding role in a previously unimagined technology.[206]

America was constantly changing, however, and the public's expectations of the business sector were ever more demanding. Thalidomide and the Dalkon Shield had raised the bar for acceptable production standards and consumer accountability. When the Medical Device Amendments became another weapon in the government's regulatory arsenal and A. H. Robins was dissolving its operations under the burden of litigation, a Houston attorney was preparing to file suit against Dow Corning, whose products had never been ruled defective.[207]

Robert Mithoff was a junior associate of the legendary Joe Jamail, who made litigation history by winning the twentieth century's largest civil damage award from Texaco—$10.5 billion— earning him the title "King of Torts." Mithoff aspired to similar fame. His client, Norma Corley, had suffered breast infections that she attributed to a ruptured implant. There was also the continuing embarrassment of silicone gel seeping from an open wound beneath one of her breasts. Several operations followed, and Mithoff claimed that but for an implant defect, all of them were unnecessary. Because Dow Corning had never lost a suit involving a breast implant, its attorneys refused all settlement offers, thus forcing a trial. The company believed it should not have to pay more than five thousand dollars, and then only to mitigate trial costs. Arguing before an engrossed panel of jurors, Mithoff claimed the manufacturers owed his client a product that was not defective. The jury agreed and awarded the plaintiff $170,000. Years later, Mithoff said ruefully, "We thought at the time it was a lot of money."[208]

In 1977, any judgment against a medical device manufacturer was a noteworthy precedent for tort lawyers. Even though Dow Corning insisted the award was excessive, it lost all subsequent appeals. Of course it did not represent a serious financial blow to the corporation, but a new era was at hand, one where a repetition of related legal actions can provoke mass tort (class action) litigation. In the case of breast implants, it would take three judgments. *Corley vs. Dow Corning* was strike one with another pitch coming.

Mithoff was not allowed to refer to the Medical Device Amendments during his arguments; the legislation was moot in a court of law because it was enacted four years after his client received her implants. Neither could Dow Corning's defense attorneys strengthen their argument by citing a successful FDA review of their product because there had never been one. Long after the device amendments, the company's strategy was to resist the agency by challenging its classification of breast implants. Dow Corning stood firm on the conviction that breast implants should be Class II because there were so many years of safe use. In step with this campaign was ASPRS, the largest plastic surgical trade organization in America. Had the plastic surgeons urged the industry to comply with the full intent of the device amendments, then the entire course of implant history might have been radically different. A full review of the product would have occurred long before consumer advocates and plaintiff attorneys attained their destructive force. But the plastic surgeons were heady with the success of a unique confrontation with the FTC. Along with Dow Corning, they stood prepared to challenge another regulatory agency.[209]

Plastic surgery's battle with the FTC had arisen over Trade Commissioner Michael Pertschuk's unprecedented stand against specialty board certification. Plastic surgeons who had completed the board certification process had long objected to claims of equivalent expertise coming from other specialties. What Pertschuk saw was the public's interest being ill-served by a contemporary guild system. He wanted to quash the specialty boards decisively and permanently. He did not strike blindly at plastic surgery, but instead he lobbed his first salvo at the AMA; not disposed to a fight, the nation's largest medical organization agreed to sign a consent decree allowing physicians to advertise without imposing an ethics violation. Pertschuk turned next to plastic surgery. Why? "We were conspicuous, we were relatively small, and they thought we represented an easy target," recalled Peter Randall, ASPRS president-elect.[210]

Refusing to capitulate as the AMA had done, ASPRS President Rex Peterson defied a 1977 subpoena demanding ASPRS records since 1946. Each member was assessed four hundred dollars to retain the services of a former FTC attorney. At risk were the high training standards of the specialty and its voluntary examining board. Led by the American Board of Surgery, every other medical and surgical board, along with deans of the nation's medical schools and presidents of state medical societies, lent their spiritual support, but it cost ASPRS a half million dollars. The FTC position was not helped when Commissioner Pertschuk agreed with a *Newsweek* reporter who suggested the relaxed standards his agency was pushing for might lead to unqualified physicians doing brain surgery. Caught on tape, the commissioner added, "but what the hell, we will finally know what is happening in the medical marketplace." When the public's outrage settled down, the FTC quietly backed away from its demands on plastic surgery.[211]

ASPRS leaders weren't as well prepared to confront the FDA as they needed to be. They were largely uninformed about the history of advancing regulatory power in America or the tragic Dalkon Shield debacle that prompted the deliberations and conclusions of the Cooper Committee. Neither could they anticipate the FDA's longstanding tradition of ignoring all lobbying efforts from professional organizations. The agency had never been granted jurisdiction over the medical profession, so its interaction with health professionals was limited to its advisory panels. ASPRS imagined that a powerful statement from a majority of plastic surgeons in America might swing the agency's position in their favor. But the FTC and the FDA were given conflicting powers by Congress, and their tactics differed as well. FDA commissioners were not in the habit of granting careless interviews to the Washington press corps. The agency's power lay in its habit of saying as little as possible and postponing decisions time and again. Neither the industry, the surgeons, the public, nor the press learned how the breast implant would be regulated until 1982, six years following enactment of the device amendments. That's when the FDA announced its intent to conduct a full review of all varieties and models of implantable silicone gel breast devices. This meant the agency was standing firm on its plan to designate breast implants as Class III devices, requiring manufacturers to supply evidence of safety and efficacy as if they were submitting a new product for approval. Furthermore, the FDA was making a distinction between the gel device and the saline-filled device, even though both were contained within a similar elastomeric sheath.

According to statutory mandate, the FDA was required to solicit written comments from the public. The ASPRS filed comments on behalf of all practicing plastic surgeons on July 1, 1982. Three arguments were offered: 1.) many thousands of women had already benefited from breast implants; 2.) breast implants had already been proved safe and remarkably free of complications; 3.) sufficient information existed to develop performance standards. But the surgeons would wait in vain for the accelerated review process they were hoping for. No reply was ever received because the FDA is not required to reply to comments and rarely does so. Neither did manufacturers know where they stood for another six years (twelve since the 1976 amendment) Then in 1988, all factions learned that manufacturers were required to file a PMAA (premarket approval application). Months would pass before deadlines were announced.[212]

While Dow Corning marked time awaiting the FDA's definition of review guidelines, it grappled with a different regulatory challenge, the use of liquid silicones for injection into soft tissues. Industrial applications for the liquid silicones were already plentiful and still multiplying. Whenever commercial products could be improved by reducing friction or eliminating foam, a silicone polymer often resolved the problem. Eventually, injectable silicones became a prospect for clinical benefits. Believing that lubricating fluids could be further refined as a soft tissue filler, Midland chemists created a polymer with a narrower range of molecules and less mineral residue. Concurrent with the introduction of this new product, Dow Corning applied the term "medical grade" to all polymers intended for subcutaneous injection or surgical implantation.

Because liquid silicones had become widely available during the postwar industrial boom, anyone could obtain them from a variety of commercial sources and use them for plausible or questionable motives. In Japan and other Asian nations where paraffin and petroleum jelly had long served as vehicles for breast enlargement, the liquid silicones gained acceptance because of their chemical stability and tissue compatibility. Liquid silicone required no activators, whether intended for industrial or for clinical applications. Yet, many unqualified users ignorant of polymer chemistry continued to add a variety of mystifying chemical adjuncts. H. D. Kagan, a Los Angeles osteopathic physician, popularized the so-called "Sakurai Method." Named for its Japanese originator who favored the inflammatory properties of chemical blends, the mixture remained in place unlike liquid silicone that tended to migrate according to the laws of gravity.[213]

Aware of these unexamined polymer uses, the FDA warned Dow Corning in writing on December 9, 1964, that "your firm must cease disseminating printed matter or other promotional material that recommends or suggests use of silicone preparations for medical purposes not covered by an approved application, and that all orders for Medical Fluid 360 must remain untitled." US marshals were later dispatched by the agency to seize product en route from Midland, Michigan, to various practitioners, among them Dr. Kagan in Los Angeles. Criminal charges were filed against Dow Corning officials for interstate shipment of an unapproved drug. Even under the 1938 revision of the food and drug act, Dow Corning was obligated to inform the agency of any evidence pertaining to the safety of silicone injections. Under the 1962 amendment, an advance determination of the product's clinical efficacy was required. Not until June 8, 1965, did Midland executives submit a "Notice of Claimed Investigation for a New Drug," accompanied by a protocol for the clinical study of DC360 liquid (for research purposes designated as MDX 4-4011 Medical Fluid). The FDA assigned ND #2707 to the product in July 1965 and began its long wait for the data Dow Corning had promised. Nine investigators were recruited: seven plastic surgeons, one otolaryngologist, and one dermatologist.[214]

At New York University, plastic surgeon Tom Rees collaborated with Donald Ballantyne, who had a PhD in animal studies of the medical fluid. Ballantyne's task was to design experiments using laboratory rats and then Rees translated investigative findings into clinical protocols using volunteer patients. Little difference was noted between DC360 Medical Fluid and the Sakurai-like formulations still popular in Japan and California. Both products were well tolerated by the recipient tissue; any inflammatory reactions observed were mild and transient. Rees concluded that liquid silicone injected conscientiously into the earliest facial wrinkles could effectively forestall the onset of an aging appearance. Dr. Franklin Ashley in Los Angeles injected the fluid into patients with Romberg's Disease, a rare but progressive wasting of the fatty layer beneath the skin surface. Treated victims were thrilled by the return of natural contour. Not yet explored were questions about the fate of injected silicone in the body. Where did it go? Was it metabolized before leaving the body? Despite the interest of physicians and patients alike, the answers remained a mystery.

Podiatrist S.W. Balkin worked with liquid silicone for many years in relative obscurity. Affiliated with the Podiatry Section at Los Angeles County University of Southern California Medical Center, he saw patients who suffered painful weight bearing because of a loss of protective plantar fat. Also common were diabetics with numb feet, leading to calluses and ulcers. Over a forty-year span (1964–2004), he treated 1,575 patients using more than twenty-five thousand injections, conservatively instilling minute quantities for the purpose of replacing focal loss of plantar fat. In 1986, he persuaded Dow Corning to sponsor a two-year clinical trial. Close follow-up showed remarkably consistent relief of symptoms, often with complete elimination of pain, and only a rare complication. Microscopic examination of selected biopsies confirmed that inflammation was minimal at all injected sites. Concurrently, a British trial of liquid silicone injected into diabetic feet was conducted at the Manchester Royal Infirmary with similar outcomes. Yet this specialized use of silicone never received FDA approval.[215]

Regulators seemed far less impressed by favorable clinical results than they were concerned about sporadic reports of indiscriminate use by charlatans. Las Vegas plastic surgeon Ed Kopf was appalled by the breast deformities he witnessed following injection of as much as a liter of silicone blended with inflammatory additives, a predicament he called "silicone mastitis." Kopf lobbied the Nevada attorney general and later the state legislature to restrict the practice and succeeded. In 1975, Nevada banned silicone injections for any medical purpose, and California amended its business and professional code listing silicone injection of a human breast as a misdemeanor offense. Given these statutory precedents, the FDA was disinclined to grant approval for any clinical application of liquid silicone. A notable exception would be its 1994 blessing of liquid silicone for replacing ocular vitreous fluid.[216]

Long before the nine Dow Corning investigators were ready to report their clinical experience, the FDA took note of deficiencies in the company's progress reports and in October 1967 suspended ND #2702. Two years later they agreed to reinstate the application. Despite receiving promise after promise, the company still couldn't retrieve enough data from its investigators. Of 1,333 patients enrolled in the original protocol, completed reports arrived from only five of nine investigators. One of them, New

York dermatologist Norman Orentreich, was treating dozens of patients for wrinkles and acne scars, indications that were excluded from the study. Following investigation, he was dropped from the panel of investigators. Realizing it was losing control of its Investigational New Drug (IND) designation, Dow Corning withdrew its application in 1976.[217]

Based on expectations that a resubmitted application would be transferred from the Bureau of Drugs to the new Bureau of Devices, Dow Corning filed again in September 1977 and succeeded. Designated as IDE 2702, injectable silicone was now a transitional Class III device instead of a drug, yet still vulnerable to agency conditions such as limiting use to severe facial deformities such as hemifacial atrophy and facial lipodystrophy. Once again, all cosmetic indications were excluded from the protocol, but Dr. Orentreich, who somehow managed to regain entry, enrolled hundreds more of his cosmetic patients.[218]

Not until August 1990 was Dow Corning prepared to file its report summarizing results of the injection protocol. The FDA promptly declared the findings unsatisfactory, citing missing photography, absence of objective measurements of improvement, and limited follow-up. Dow Corning had reached the end of its patience and so had the FDA. When additional studies of safety and efficacy were demanded by the agency, the company elected not to respond. Their Investigational Device Exemption (IDE) lapsed in January 1992, twenty-seven years after its initial submission. Long before any controversy arose over silicone breast implants, the FDA had experienced ample frustration dealing with Dow Corning and vice versa. The company's frustration, however, was born of its own clinical investigators unwillingness to maintain precise records required by a regulatory agency that meant business.

Twelve years into their Los Angeles cancer study, Dennis Deapen and Garry Brody persevered to maintain eligibility for enough patients to permit valid data collection. Although thirty-five hundred patients were initially enrolled, there were now only 3,111 who retained the necessary local residence. Not until 1986 were they prepared to make an initial calculation of comparative cancer risks. Based on 18,476 person-years of implant exposure, they found no increase in breast cancer incidence. Neither had implants served as a diagnostic barrier to early detection of cancers. Already apparent was a reduction in breast cancer incidence among the implanted group, but because it was not statistically significant, they chose not to feature the tumor-sparing effect.[219]

By inference, the data presented was important for predictive reasons. The investigators already knew that breast implants could not be the sole cause of breast cancer; women had contracted the disease for centuries, and most women with breast cancer did not have breast implants. Furthermore, it was clear that all but very few women with exposure to silicone gel were cancer-free. Given investigators' results so far, the prospect of a cancer epidemic resulting from breast implants was, at best, fanciful. At worst, silicone might serve as a contributing factor (cofactor). The question then was whether any association would be a weak one or a strong one like smoking and lung cancer? The USC data demonstrated conclusively that any possible link would be extremely weak.

An independent epidemiologist provided a critique of the Los Angeles study, declaring it an excellent first step. The design was well conceived and carefully conducted, but it needed additional years of follow-up for a final answer. The database deserved to be maintained for a reading in five more years, with a focus on women over forty with a higher expected risk of breast cancer.[220]

The study's investigators agreed with a need to revisit the question when their database could display more statistical power. Dow Corning's management was pleased to learn that silicone gel was not proving to be a human carcinogen, and offered twenty-five thousand dollars to keep the study running. Meanwhile, the company was facing another liability challenge, one that would dwarf Corley vs. Dow Corning in financial impact and legal significance.[221]

In 1982, Maria Stern met with plaintiff attorney Nancy Hersh and voiced her complaint: a ruptured implant found by her surgeon and replaced with a device provided by Dow Corning at no cost. In the attorney's view, the company had already admitted fault by offering a free implant. But Hersh wasn't as interested in the rupture as she was in Stern's complaints of chronic fatigue and migratory joint pains. Stern theorized that the silicone was spreading throughout the body and found a doctor who without any confirming evidence agreed with her. Hersh even conjured a link between silicone and illnesses affecting other women. The legwork was delegated to her new associate, Dan Bolton, a recent law school graduate who had never before handled a product liability case but welcomed the challenge. A search revealed a precedent for unexplained arthritis and fatigue among Asian women with silicone injected into their breasts. Hersh took the offensive and petitioned for disclosure of documents that might be pertinent to the case. A judge ruled that Dow Corning must open its files. So Dan Bolton was sent to Midland, flying first class at the expense of the company. Confident of its position and not yet aware of what was in store, Dow Corning also paid the attorney's hotel charges.[222]

Bolton was given full access to corporate files during a visit lasting several days. He went about his task not as a scientist would—looking for all evidence pertinent to the issues—but rather as a lawyer should, selecting only documents that supported his client's position. For example, there were letters from salesmen in the field who, because they knew little about prior research, implied there hadn't been any. Ignoring decades of published data, Bolton pictured himself convincing a jury there was no research assuring safety. Despite many studies of gel bleed, he believed he had uncovered a hidden problem: leakage of silicone from the gel implant surface. Ignoring the favorable toxicology studies conducted by Dow Chemical in 1948, Bolton focused on a letter from Dr. John Heggers of the University of Chicago soliciting funds for studying the role of immunity in capsule contraction. Dow Corning had turned him down and Bolton wondered why? Departing with eight hundred documents in his briefcase, he was convinced he held the smoking gun needed to win his client's case.[223]

Preparing for trial early in 1985, Hersh and Bolton found experts willing to offer personal theories about how silicone might produce an immune system disorder. One of them, Marc Lappe, taught bioethics instead of immunology and didn't believe it unethical to offer opinions about immunologic diseases. Remarkably, defense attorneys failed to limit the scope of Lappe's testimony. By this time, Bolton was a true believer, convinced that breast implants caused autoimmune disease, a term he featured at the proceedings. Dow Corning's defense attorneys were prepared to offer a pretrial settlement; they could anticipate the sympathy the plaintiff would surely elicit, also the confusion that jurors might experience sorting complex medical testimony. Confident they held a winning hand, Hersh and Bolton refused all offers. And they were right.[224]

The jury awarded Mrs. Stern two hundred and eleven thousand dollars for her pain and suffering and another one and a half million in punitive damages, indicating that the manufacturer deserved punishment for its wrongful actions. Hersh later admitted she should have asked for much more. Witnesses for the defense had failed to disabuse the jury of the folly inherent in Lappe's testimony. Never presented were studies showing silicone's negligible immune responsiveness. What Hersh and Bolton had achieved was convincing a judge and jury that a disease had occurred for which there was no diagnostic proof but that the company was to blame. All that Dow Corning attorneys could get from the judge was an immediate surrender of Bolton's incriminating documents and a gag order. Their contents could not be discussed publicly based on the company's argument that they were not representative of the entire body of knowledge about silicone implantable devices. Stern vs. Dow Corning was not only a defeat but also a legal tour de force. The largest producer of silicone medical products was two strikes down and still at bat.

In 1988, two very public moments brought sudden attention to the possibility that serious risks might follow breast implantation. In the June issue of Ms. magazine, Sybil Norden Goldrich described for a national audience of feminists the terror

of "enduring amputations of both breasts for cancer, then suffering five failed operations . . . and countless days of pain and
worry," all because of silicone breast implants. Despite promises
of a successful reconstruction, her breasts first hardened, then
moved, and then became infected time and again. In the end, she
was no closer to anatomic restoration than when she started. "All I
ended up with were more scars," she added. Her article elicited an
avalanche of letters and telephone calls from women who felt similarly violated. Then in October 1988, Sidney Wolfe announced on
CNN that, according to evidence recently made available to Public
Citizen, an epidemic of breast cancer would soon befall women
who had submitted to silicone gel breast implants. He cited animal studies paid for and then hidden by Dow Corning because
they confirmed silicone's carcinogenic role. Nowhere in his warning did he acknowledge existence of the USC study showing that
women with breast implants were no more vulnerable, perhaps
less vulnerable, to breast cancer.[225]

Still smarting from a judgment ten times the cost of their
first loss in court, and for a product that represented less than 1
percent of its total revenue, Dow Corning continued to think of
itself both as pioneer and standard-bearer for silicone medical
product innovation. Its research and development budget was
unmatched in the industry, and its marketing programs were as
energetic as they had always been. But there were lingering doubts
among Midland managers about prospects for the mammary
device. Dow Corning's representative to the FDA's Advisory Panel
for General and Plastic Surgery, Art Rathjen, continued to monitor
discussions in Washington and provide company executives with
summaries and transcripts. Since the 1970s and early 1980s when
the panel was dominated by practicing surgeons largely in awe of
the devices available, the sentiments of the group had changed
dramatically. Its new chairman was Norman Anderson, whose
specialty was internal medicine, not surgery. He had no experience implanting any medical device. His responsibilities at Johns
Hopkins Medical Center were more administrative than clinical. Furthermore, he was an outspoken critic of any woman who

would submit to surgery for any cosmetic motive. Whenever that surgery involved silicone breast implants, he held that the devices should be devoid of all risk. The FDA's executive secretary for the panel was Paul Tilton, who was already familiar with the challenge of monitoring and regulating silicone products. For years he had managed Dow Corning's problematic liquid silicone application.

When Anderson convened a meeting of the advisory panel in November 1988, Tilton had arranged for on-site television coverage and invited participation from several individuals the panel had not previously heard from. They included Sybil Goldrich, speaking for her newly formed Command Trust Network (CTN); Sidney Wolfe, representing Public Citizen; bioethicist and recent trial expert Marc Lappe, and attorney Dan Bolton, who was not yet finished with Dow Corning. Sitting near the back of the room was Denise Dunleavy, a New York City attorney whose client had developed not one but two cancers following breast reconstruction with a polyurethane-coated device. The entire scene, according to returning emeritus panel chairman J. B. Lynch, looked like it had been carefully staged by the agency to send a new message about the fate of breast implants.[226]

Anderson introduced Robert Sheridan, director of the Office of Device Evaluation, who enumerated the many regulatory hoops through which the breast implant must pass. He was followed by Nirmal Mishra, D.V.M., who offered what seemed a laundry list of FDA concerns that left many present wondering whether he had bothered to review decades of prior silicone research or even the preceding fourteen years of device panel deliberations. His accounting of contraction and leakage omitted the important electron microscopic studies of Rudolph and Abraham. His discussion of cancer risk was limited to rat studies and ignored recent clinical data. During the limited time offered to Dow Corning representative Robert Rylee tried to fill the gaps left by Dr. Mishra, making available to panel doctors Gerhard Brand and Garry Brody to place in perspective expressed concerns about cancer risk. Brand, a professor at the University of Minnesota and recognized tumor biologist, discounted any clinical applicability

of solid state carcinogenesis, believing that silicone was a biologically insignificant example of the phenomenon. Brody spoke for
plastic surgeons: "We are equally concerned when our patients
are unduly alarmed by scare headlines and extrapolation of animal data that is meaningless in humans."

Sybil Goldrich was so taken by the opportunity to tell her
story before a government-sponsored committee that she couldn't
stop talking. Finally asked by Dr. Anderson to summarize, she
offered copies of her *Ms.* article to anyone desiring one and finally
sat down. Sidney Wolfe bounded to the microphone and asked
whether he might preface his planned remarks with an observation. Without waiting for a reply, he delivered a broadside at
several professional surgical associations for their organized
resistance to the proposed Medical Device Amendments in 1976.
No evidence was offered or later revealed that any such boycott
had taken place. Then he tried to refute Dr. Brand by declaring
that "animals are the best route we have for predicting and preventing human cancer. Only animal studies can predict whether
or not cancer will occur in humans," a statement that would have
delighted Congressman Delaney but horrified any cancer epidemiologist listening. Ignoring or perhaps just unaware that inbred
mice develop tumors only because of their genetically weakened
state, he pleaded for the panel to accept only animal data, a position he has not since relinquished. Television reporters awaited
adjournment so they might give Dr. Wolfe and his sound bites
plenty of broadcast exposure.

Marc Lappe deftly skipped past the fact that he was neither a
physician nor a biomaterials scientist and embarked on a lengthy
discussion of clinical risks from medical devices in general.
Accusing Cronin and Gerow of reckless haste in their development of the mammary device, he offered his own solution: many
more years of development without Dow Corning's participation.
He placed no faith in corporate-financed research, omitting where
he thought funding for product innovation should come from.

Dan Bolton proceeded to feature testimony heard during
Stern vs. Dow Corning without visible concern about violating the

judge's gag order. Based on what he characterized as his "scientific review of the evidence," Bolton called for immediate removal of
breast implants from the marketplace. Turning to Dow Corning's
representatives, he demanded release of all court-protected documents. Suspecting that Bolton might be overstepping court orders,
Chairman Anderson cautioned him about use of such strong language. Television reporters descended on Bolton at the next break.

Sitting before her television that evening in San Francisco,
Mariann Hopkins was flipping channels when she heard Goldrich
relate a personal story of suffering similar to her own. Later she
said, "at the time, I thought I was the only person who suffered
problems with my implants." Pausing to hear more, she heard
an attorney from her own city tell a national audience that breast
implants were unsafe and should be removed from the market.
The next day, she called Bolton's office for an appointment. One
week later, he filed the third complaint against Dow Corning on
behalf of Hopkins. The outcome of her trial would launch breast
implant awards into the stratosphere.[227]

Following the 1988 hearing in Washington, voting members of the panel deliberated privately for hours. They were not of
a mind to remove mammary devices from the marketplace, but
there was unanimous conviction that the industry must provide
a full disclosure of all it knew about the devices. Panelists recognized bias and emotionalism when they saw it, and they knew
how ridiculous it was for a plaintiff attorney to issue scientific pro-
nouncements. But they also doubted the sincerity of Dow Corning,
given reports of suppressed documents believed fraudulent in a
courtroom.[228]

At the time of the 1988 hearing, most plastic surgeons were
busy caring for their patients, and except for a few, were not alert
to government concerns about silicone devices. They were later
blamed for ignoring complications altogether, but as early as 1982,
a committee of The American Society for Aesthetic Plastic Surgery
(ASAPS), a trade group made up of plastic surgeons whose practices are predominately cosmetic, was paying close attention to
incidents such as deflation and rupture. Members knew these

were uncommon occurrences from their own clinical experience, but they sought means for earlier detection and encouraged efforts to reduce the risk. Meanwhile, Dr. Rudolph had addressed microdroplet leakage, Dr. Brody had inaugurated the study to answer the cancer question, and the panel under Dr. Lynch's leadership had for several years conducted an organized surveillance of complications as they were reported. But to a new and biased panel chairman and a demonstrably risk-averse FDA, reassurances about breast implants were not what they were looking for. Consumer advocates, the press, and the plaintiff's bar were all on high alert, and communications technology was moving at a faster pace than new evidence was coming in from systematic clinical studies required to answer the remaining difficult questions.[229]

Although busy enough with his own administrative responsibilities, FDA Commissioner Frank Young took time to respond to Public Citizen accusations of impropriety. Responding directly to Sidney Wolfe, he summarized results of the agency's review of the Dow Corning animal studies, including consultation with recognized cancer authorities who believed the kinds of tumors seen were unlikely to occur in humans, leading his agency to conclude that "no compelling evidence supports a banning regulation." That the letter's content was ignored by Public Citizen is apparent from the media frenzy that followed. That this scientifically responsible letter and its conclusions would be disregarded by the time Dr. Kessler took charge is both unfortunate and inexcusable.[230]

In July 1989, plastic surgeons representing ASPRS and its research affiliate, PSEF, met in Santa Barbara with representatives of the major silicone product manufacturers. The discussion was entirely devoted to the expanding list of alleged silicone health risks. Difficult to explain was the focus on breast implants when everyone present knew the very same polymers were used to fabricate hundreds of silicone medical products. Equally confounding was the sudden appearance of problems after nearly three decades of presumably safe use. Surgeons in attendance knew of the hostility directed at Dow Corning for its apparent withholding of evidence. When asked to explain the company's posture, Robert

Rylee initially sidestepped the question, citing the San Francisco judge's gag order, but later explained that the carcinogenesis data featured by Sidney Wolfe was proprietary, meaning his company had contracted with an Arizona firm to repeat the Oppenheimer solid state carcinogenesis experiments, it owned the data, and it deserved to retain it for its own use. Yet, the findings hadn't varied from the original results. Why then had Dow Corning not been entirely forthcoming with the FDA? "It is not our policy to inform the FDA of anything we are not required by law to tell them," quipped Rylee.[231]

But the agency already knew about a 25 percent incidence of tumors in the particular rat species selected for study. Public Citizen received word of the experiments from an FDA staff member who was unaware of a biologic precedent for this kind of neoplasia. Sidney Wolfe was clever enough to make it all seem like Dow Corning was hiding experimental results never before revealed to the scientific community.

The impression Rylee left with plastic surgeons assembled in Santa Barbara, however, was that protecting his company's marketplace dominance was more important than releasing scientific data in a timely manner. Some present wondered whether Dow Corning understood that protecting the company's market share was no longer as important as preserving its integrity.

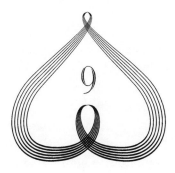

SILICONE DISEASE?
OR SILICONE
VICTIMIZATION!

"This isn't just about breast implants;
this is about the empowerment of women!"
—Sybil Goldrich[232]

W hen Sybil Goldrich addressed the readership of *Ms,* the immensely successful publication for women, and spoke candidly about her personal problems with ruptured breast implants, she delivered a galvanizing message to an audience that was both politically sophisticated and demonstrably proactive. Many were personally exposed to silicone devices, and many more were acquainted with women who had experienced implant surgery. Goldrich, a Beverly Hills homemaker and wife of a surgeon, was medically informed herself, knew how to search medical journals for information, and wasn't bashful about asking penetrating questions. She was also a quick study on the parameters of medical device regulation. For example, she knew that medical devices had not been effectively regulated until 1976, fourteen years after silicone breast implants were first used. She informed her readers that although the FDA had not yet ruled on the safety of silicone gel, it had declared in 1982 that "breast implants present a potentially unreasonable risk of injury." That sounded like a warning to her, and she sounded a trumpet like none heard before.

Goldrich also learned that in 1985 the FDA had initiated a program called Medical Device Reporting (MDR) and that manufacturers were required to submit any report of an implantable device failure. Agency staff told her that compliance with this requirement was poor, so she did something about that. Her article closed with a plea to readers: report directly to the FDA any problem you or a friend might have experienced with a breast implant. *Ms* editors obliged the author by listing the address and phone number of MDR in Rockville, MD. For weeks thereafter, the phone didn't stop ringing at the agency; mail volume was unprecedented in MDR's short history.[233]

Mrs. Goldrich's Beverly Hills mailbox also filled up most days with correspondence from readers expressing their own disappointment. She collected dozens of stories from women whose implants had "become hardened or misshapen or changed position" just as she had reported. And she received a flood of letters from those who had read for the first time that a leaking implant might cause autoimmune diseases such as rheumatoid arthritis, scleroderma, even lupus. Goldrich heard from people whose words echoed her own fury, among them Kathryn Anneken of Louisville, Kentucky. The course of both women's lives changed permanently after they established the Command Trust Network (CTN), at first a clearinghouse for breast implant information but in time a powerful consumer force in regulatory politics. Theirs wouldn't be the only assembly of like-minded women; there would be many others. Few would admit they had once acted on the basis of a strong motivation for breast surgery; instead, they responded with anger because of what they believed had been done without full disclosure of risks. But were their ailments real or imagined?

What Sybil Goldrich and others were in the process of identifying was a numerator, an approximation of the number of patients who were experiencing problems. What had not yet been assessed was the much larger denominator, every woman with breast implants. Estimates ranged from one to two million women. Missing altogether was knowledge of what percentage of women were experiencing health issues and whether or not their implants played any role. What was certain was that, within a short time, Goldrich and Anneken had successfully mobilized a select group of "fightin' mad women," as one observer described them, some with real problems and many more with fear of impending tragedy. Left off their agenda for the time being was any consideration of the broader population of men and women with other silicone exposures, but that time would come. CTN would later publicize warnings to diabetics everywhere that syringes lubricated with silicone were dangerous and should be outlawed.[234]

Although the risk of systemic illnesses was not initially featured by Ms. Goldrich, she eventually informed her worried audience that a threat of autoimmune disease loomed larger than any cancer risk. Her visits to the Medline database and to medical libraries uncovered case reports appearing in medical journals. In 1964, Miyoshi and associates first suggested that a foreign substance injected into a woman's breast might lead to symptoms involving the joints, the muscles, and the skin—in other words, the very tissues that held the body together. These were collectively known as connective tissue diseases, and because they were thought to be the result of immunity to one's own body, the term autoimmune disease was applied to the same disorders.

Miyoshi also reported that a blend of paraffin and silicone injected into the breasts of two young women led to elevations in gamma globulin, a blood protein involved in immunity. One patient improved after the foreign material was removed, leading the author to speculate that the injected material was functioning as an adjuvant, a substance that exaggerates an immune reaction.

Thus another name was introduced, "human adjuvant disease," presumably because there was precedent in the animal kingdom. Rats are known to develop arthritis following adjuvant injections. But no one had ever witnessed a similar condition in humans. Nevertheless, belief in its existence proved durable throughout the years of the breast implant controversy.[235]

Miyoshi's theory was revisited in 1973 when Yoshida reported seven more women with intermittent fever and joint pain following breast enlargement using injected foreign materials. He also likened the affliction to a human adjuvant effect even though symptoms hadn't developed until thirteen years following the injections. In four of seven patients, symptoms were relieved by removal of the offending material. Several more reports prompted Yasao Kumagai to collect thirty similar cases in 1979. Unique to this report were four patients with classic signs of progressive systemic sclerosis (scleroderma), a connective tissue disease characterized by stiffened body surfaces. Not one of these had received silicone; instead, they had been injected with "Organagen," a processed petroleum jelly. So far, there was no consistent pattern of disease, no common latency period, and no similarity of the offending agent. Another physician, Hirobumi Kondo, added nine more cases to the total and began to think like an epidemiologist. Estimating that ten thousand women in Japan had received injections to enlarge their breasts since 1962 and knowing that the expected incidence of scleroderma in Japanese women was 2.46 per million, he concluded that nine cases in a small population segment was enough to identify a condition specific to women receiving illicit breast injections. Yet, most of his patients had received either paraffin or petroleum jelly; only two had received silicone fluid. There was still no pattern to Kondo's "new disease."[236]

In America, clinical reports of a similar kind were rarer still; the use of paraffin, petroleum jelly and even liquid silicone for breast enlargement was uncommon because the Cronin implant had dominated augmentation mammaplasty since 1962. If problems similar to those reported in Japan were to appear anywhere else in the world, two likely prospects were Las Vegas and Tijuana, Mexico, where injecting materials into breasts was more commonly pursued. But the victims of silicone mastitis in both cities had never complained of rheumatic or immune disorders nor have they since.[237]

On the other hand, two noteworthy reports came first from a Boston plastic surgeon and later from three immunologists in Sydney, Australia. In 1977, Dr. Barry Uretsky's Boston patient developed a high fever and diffuse joint pain within twenty-four hours of breast implantation. In fact, she was so sick that he felt obliged to remove the implants without delay, and she recovered promptly. Uretsky concluded that the implants must have played a causative role. Then in 1982, Sheryl van Nunen, Paul Gatenby, and Anthony Basten encountered three patients who developed connective tissue diseases two to three years after silicone gel implants. Each woman's medical diagnosis differed from the others'. No laboratory studies indicated that silicone was the offending agent. Their manuscript was submitted to *Arthritis and Rheumatism*, the leading American journal for rheumatologic diseases. Without a uniform diagnosis, the authors elected to use the unsubstantiated term "human adjuvant disease." Their manuscript was rejected, but the editor later chose to publish it for the purpose of eliciting similar experiences. The appearance of this report in a prominent journal prompted a deluge of similar accounts from physicians treating women with a prior history of breast implantation.[238]

Two of these physicians were Steven Weiner at UCLA and Michael Weisman at UCSD. They would develop opposing positions regarding the relationship between silicone and connective tissue disease, largely because they chose different methods of study. Weiner started with three patients experiencing pains affecting several joints (polyarthropathy) but none with the diagnostic criteria for any recognized connective tissue disease. The interval between breast augmentation and the onset of symptoms varied from one to four years. Flimsy evidence notwithstanding, Dr. Weiner proposed a causal link specific to the gel device. Soon, his Los Angeles practice attracted many more women with breast implants and unexplained joint pains, serving to confirm his convictions about silicone.[239]

Dr. Weisman, on the other hand, was more the skeptic. He understood that the number of women with augmented breasts was increasing, especially in Southern California, where as many as one in one hundred might have received implants. He was an experienced rheumatologist who knew that episodic reporting of joint pain was commonplace, especially in an aging but physically active population. Rheumatoid arthritis, the most common connective tissue disease, afflicts one patient in a thousand, many more of them women than men. Taking into account all connective tissue diseases, the prevalence is closer to one in a hundred. Combining these ratios, he determined there might be ten thousand in every million women with concurrent breast implants and rheumatic disease. So Weisman's speculation was that the alleged association might be nothing more than coincidental occurrence. For a test of his theory, he adopted a retrospective cohort study model that required access to a population of breast implant recipients. Thomas Vecchione, a San Diego plastic surgeon who had previously contributed specimens for Dr. Rudolph's gel bleed studies, was again willing to enlist support from several of his colleagues.

Their task was to review the medical records for patients seeking augmentation mammaplasty between 1970 and 1984, then ask permission to distribute a questionnaire inquiring about late complications, and finally request a medical examination if rheumatic symptoms were reported. Personal contact with each surgeon guaranteed privacy. There were 378 women available for record review, but only 125 returned their questionnaires and accepted follow-up phone calls. Because people experiencing problems are more likely to respond to studies of this kind, Weisman believed that any possible bias favored the identification of patients with rheumatic illness. Mean duration of implant exposure among responders was 6.8 years. No patient reported symptoms indicative of any recognized rheumatic disease or features remotely suggestive of the imagined human adjuvant disease. Thirty-eight patients who reported joint pains were found to be either recovering from traumatic injuries or experiencing degenerative arthritis consistent with their age. Based on Weisman's calculation of the expected frequency of the rheumatic illnesses, he concluded that augmentation mammaplasty was unlikely to cause any connective tissue disease. Although the study was small, Weisman had shown that all symptoms reported could be explained as a coincidental occurrence.[240]

As with the Los Angeles breast cancer study, Weisman's investigation was declared useless by all who devoutly accepted a link between silicone and rheumatic disease. Neither did 125 patients followed for seven years qualify for an epidemiologist's validation. Yet reasonable people looking at the question objectively could infer from the findings that any possible association between silicone and disease had to be a weak one. Most rheumatologists knew that women were predisposed to rheumatic disorders. And most women with breast implants were not experiencing symptoms of autoimmune disease. But these were facts better handled by biostatisticians than by fear mongers.

Despite differences in their approach to the problem, Dr. Weiner's accounting of three patients with unexplained arthritic pain created much more of a public stir than Dr. Weisman's thirty-eight patients with understandable joint pains. Sybil Goldrich made certain that her Command Trust Network following knew they should seek Dr. Weiner's counsel at UCLA and avoid Dr. Weisman at UCSD. Meanwhile, editors of medical journals throughout the nation were receiving an avalanche of manuscripts, most of them single-case reports describing a wide variety of illnesses experienced by women with breast implants. Many were published without seriously considering the possibility of coincidental occurrence.[241]

Few saw the irony: beyond our shores a variety of injected materials were supposed to cause a single ill-defined illness while Americans exposed to a single putative toxin were believed vulnerable to a medley of disorders. The mania for attributing illnesses to breast implants went beyond the rheumatic diseases and included blood disorders such as anemia and leukemia, cardiovascular diseases such as hypertension and heart attacks, lung diseases such as asthma, and extremely rare diseases such as sarcoidosis. Everyday problems such as periodontal disease and migraine headache were blamed on silicone. Critical editorial interpretation by editors of newspapers or medical journals was a scarce commodity. Few editorial writers asked why a toxic reaction took a quarter century to make its first clinical appearance. And the biggest mystery remained: why weren't all other exposures to the polymer equally poisonous? Nobody was offering plausible answers.

Far too many were so deeply invested in the controversy they stopped listening to anyone with contradictory evidence. Sidney Wolfe, who admired the energy displayed by Sybil Goldrich's following, went farther faster than she had dared. Nothing short of a federally imposed removal of all breast implants from global commerce would suit him. It was never clear what he wanted for women with implants already in place. CTN relished its collaboration with Dr. Wolfe; he brought to their campaign acknowledgment of their fears and a proven record. That he came with dubious scientific credentials mattered little.

Sidney Wolfe thought of himself as a scientist who sacrificed a distinguished career in medical research in favor of a more significant public advocacy role in society. His father was an inspector for the Labor Department who repeatedly warned his son of hazards in the workplace. Wolfe aspired to a career in chemical engineering until he took a summer job in a chemical plant and came home with hydrofluoric acid burns. Instead of acting to better protect himself, he blamed the company, quit his job, and transferred his interests to medical research. After graduating from Western Reserve School of Medicine in 1965, he interrupted an internal medicine residency to serve his military obligation in Bethesda, Maryland, as a clinical associate for the National Institute of Arthritis and Metabolic Diseases. As an NIH fellow, he realized that medical research was not his cup of tea because laboratory findings couldn't be translated into public policy fast enough to suit him. He wanted action, meaning political action. He found it evenings and weekends volunteering for Ralph Nader, who epitomized his vision of a public servant. After joining Public Citizen he formed Health Research Group (HRG), a misnomer because it has never conducted research that would meet peer review standards. Accused by an interviewer of being, "confrontational, denunciatory, and uncompromising," Wolfe smiled: "That's me. We have hordes of people who are willing to compromise. The world needs more people [like me] who won't compromise." Nader once observed, "If Sid thinks you're selling out, you're off his Rolodex."[242]

In 1986, he targeted Simethicone (molecular structure not unlike silicone) as an unnecessary adulterant. Not so, according to gastroenterologists who recognized its effectiveness as an anti-flatulent. "Who needs it?" countered Wolfe, a common rejoinder of his. In many ways, Wolfe shared Harvey Washington Wiley's authoritarian traits. His later assault on saccharin, like Wiley's a century before, didn't go anywhere, but his campaign against Red Dye #2, safely used for centuries and known as amaranth, was more successful. Exploiting the cherished Delaney Clause, Wolfe relied on a single Russian study showing carcinogenic properties when the dye was administered to laboratory animals in high doses. Red Dye #2 remains banned today.[243]

While Wolfe's staff was at work on a new publication, *Women's Health Alert,* in which the breast implant chapter was famously titled, "Ticking Time Bombs," Sybil Goldrich and Kathryn Anneken were struggling to keep up with their mail, always replying to queries and testimonials with pleas for additional financial support. They established the "Breast Implant Information Network" (B.I.I.N), and assigned priority to anyone with new claims of distress or illness following breast implanta-tion. In a confounding twist of her own brand of logic, Goldrich urged her followers "to make sure the rumors you believe are true." She promised supporters that donations would be spent on "the kind of public relations efforts needed to convert rumors into doctrine." At their national meetings, guest speakers were drawn from the ranks of those who supported a link between silicone and a growing spectrum of infirmities. Lawyers and federal regulators and sympathetic television personalities made themselves available. Marc Lappe, the nonphysician ethicist with imagined immunologic expertise, was a favorite. Videotapes of these meetings were sold widely. A one-page checklist was enclosed with CTN's mailed literature, always asking for new complaints but never asking whether previously reported symptoms had resolved.[244]

Another kind of support network, Reach to Recovery, was formed by the American Cancer Society for women with breast cancer. Before reliable techniques for surgical reconstruction of a breast were developed, Reach to Recovery's mission was to persuade women to accept their deformity and live in harmony with a missing breast, be fitted with an external prosthesis, and wear a full range of fashions including bathing suits if desired. Reach to Recovery initially took no position on the implant controversy, but other breast cancer support agencies like the Y-Me National Organization for Breast Cancer soon recognized that false exaggerations of implant risk might put barriers in the path of breast reconstruction following mastectomy, perhaps even discourage early detection efforts as well. Sandy Finestone, a Reach to Recovery counselor at Hoag Hospital in Newport Beach, California, didn't wait for the American Cancer Society to define its position. She formed the Women's Implant Information Network (W.I.I.N.) for the purpose of presenting a more balanced view of the controversy. Having enjoyed all her science courses in high school, she was comfortable reading the science news. Trained as an accountant, she carefully scrutinized the numbers offered by journalists. A lot about the silicone scare didn't ring true for her. W.I.I.N.'s newsletter therefore presented both sides of the controversy. She was appalled by the silicone coverage in the *Orange County Register* and the *Los Angeles Times*. She later recalled a conversation with an *LA Times* editor who "condescended to inform me that good news doesn't sell."[245]

Prophets of toxic peril often invoke an ailing immune system to explain symptoms that are not easily categorized or given a precise diagnosis. Like the intricate blood clotting system, immunity is dependent on dozens of participating components. These include circulating cells called lymphocytes, as well as protein molecules called antibodies, both capable of becoming sensitized in order to react aggressively against foreign invaders called antigens. When in the 1790s an English family practitioner named Edward Jenner inoculated children with a harmless cowpox extract, his intent was to summon the body's production of antibodies to smallpox, a related disease. And in the 1950s, when pioneering surgeons tried to sustain the function of transplanted kidneys, they prevented organ rejection with drugs that suppressed immune function.

Blood tests for detecting immune diseases became a favored game for the activists. Independent diagnostic laboratories in Southern California recognized an opportunity to financially exploit the breast implant controversy. Alleged victims of silicone were encouraged to submit blood samples and pay large fees to confirm that their immune system had been compromised; all takers were told their results were abnormal. A Memphis laboratory based its diagnostic strategy on using silicon dioxide crystals (silica) as the stimulus for test reactions. Any variance from normal was attributed to silicone, not silica. Subjective symptoms such as fatigue, memory loss, and aching joints were attributed to a weakening of immune capacity. A growing fear of silicone and concurrent reports of a human adjuvant disease played well for all whose goals were to nurture widespread implant anxiety and ban the devices. The College of American Pathologists and the FDA issued warnings that laboratory assays claiming a silicone disease were not based on valid science.[246]

In the 1980s, immunotoxicology studies were conducted by Virginia Commonwealth University toxicologists Kimber White and Albert Munson under the auspices of the National Toxicology Program with funding from NIH. Measurement of host resistance to bacteria over the course of one-third of a test animal's lifetime revealed no influence on immunity by silicone or any silicone-containing product. These findings were later made available to the FDA.[247]

Nir Kossovsky, a pathologist at UCLA where so many "silicone cripples" were seen and treated, developed his own assay for detecting what he chose to call silicone-protein complexes circulating in the bloodstream of women with breast implants. After patenting the technique as Detecsil, he established an independent company to perform the assay commercially. A number of samples were sent to him from the Scripps Clinic in La Jolla, California, described as coming from women suspected of a silicone-related disorder. All tested positive whether or not breast implants were involved. Never able to secure FDA validation of his methods, Kossovsky instead received an FDA warning to cease his testing. Nonetheless, he was concurrently welcomed as an agency consultant and later selected to serve as a plaintiff's expert witness.[248]

While most implant critics continued to push the immune disease theory, a Houston neurologist, Bernard Patten, decided that breast implants were responsible for disorders affecting the nervous system. His evidence was based on nerve and muscle specimens. His associate, Britta Ostermeyer-Shoaib, tabulated data from one hundred women with implants; Patten alone interpreted the biopsies. There were no comparisons with control patients. Yet the news sent another wave of fear through the ranks of implant recipients. Plaintiff attorneys were delighted to add another category of disease to those already claimed for breast implants. His findings were never confirmed. To the contrary, neuropathologist Neil Rosenberg in his own institution was so appalled that he publicly refuted the doctor's biopsy readings in a paper titled "Neuromythology of Silicone Breast Implants." Patten never retracted his belief in "silicone neuropathic diseases"; neither would he submit to testimony under oath.[249]

Meanwhile, the silicone controversy had not yet attracted the full notice of plastic surgeons. Contrary to a common misconception, only very few of the 3,620 board certified surgeons who practiced both reconstructive and cosmetic surgery in 1988 were dependent on breast augmentation for their livelihood. Plastic surgeons were still called to emergency rooms for repair of traumatic injuries. They were summoned by pediatricians to initiate correction of birth defects affecting 1–2 percent of newborn infants. Cosmetic surgery often represented less than half of the average plastic surgeon's practice in the 1980s. On average, breast surgery represented 10 percent of plastic surgery procedures. So far, rheumatic complaints were coming from a limited segment of the breast implant population. And so it became the duty of the ASPRS to inform its members of an evolving regulatory bias.[250]

Newsletters provided accounts of hearings in Washington, but the busy practitioner spends less time with informal publications than with reputable journals. *Plastic and Reconstructive Surgery* (PRS) also informed its readers of proliferating allegations directed against silicone, even summarizing reports appearing in other journals such as *Arthritis and Rheumatism*. The polymer had earned its reputation for biologic safety over the span of nearly four decades, not only with plastic surgeons but neurosurgeons, orthopedic surgeons, and urologic surgeons as well. A case for existence of a health hazard was not an easy sell to surgeons of any stripe who used silicone devices with predictable success.

George Reading and Frank Thorne, the respective presidents of ASPRS and PSEF, had been alerted in 1988 to the trouble that might lie ahead for patients and their surgeons. Reading had attended the chaotic November 1988 meeting of the FDA advisory panel. At the completion of the Santa Barbara meeting held with industry representatives in July 1989, they appointed a committee charged with examining every allegation of toxicity directed against silicone, not just the gel format used for breast implants but also the elastomers used for facial reconstruction. Fourteen surgeons were appointed, all of them affiliated with academic institutions. As well-meaning as the gesture appeared, it was too little and too late. Members were committed to their own teaching responsibilities and clinical practices, and so the pace of this committee's inquiries would never catch up with a political snow-ball that never stopped rolling.

While assembled in Chicago, the committee met with Philip Cole, an epidemiologist with the University of Alabama. Cancer and connective tissue disease were the two main questions, and a full half-day was devoted to each. Cole agreed that clinical studies were better for answering questions than any animal study. The Los Angeles County cohort at fourteen years was still insufficient for a final answer. Another cohort study was needed, ideally from a different geographic region. Nothing confirms one study more convincingly than another with similar findings.[251]

Determining whether silicone was a cofactor in the development of rheumatic diseases was the greater challenge. Cancer is a yes-or-no proposition; a woman either has breast cancer or she doesn't. On the other hand, diagnostic criteria for the autoimmune disorders are highly subjective. Committees of rheumatologists meet periodically to discuss diagnostic parameters. Furthermore, the manifestations of rheumatic disease evolve slowly over the course of years. Dr. Cole couldn't help discouraging the committee when he estimated that decades might pass before the question was resolved.

Looking back, what was overlooked at this meeting was the existence of three established databases, one at the University of Alberta in Canada, another at the Mayo Clinic, and a third maintained by the Harvard School of Public Health. In Alberta, every woman with breast implants was listed on the university clinic's computer. The Mayo Clinic had long maintained health records for patients treated in surrounding Olmsted County, Minnesota. Harvard had recruited a population of nurses willing to join longitudinal drug studies. Given appropriate epidemiologic supervision, each cohort represented an opportunity to put new questions to a test. More time would pass before these databases were made available to answer questions about silicone safety.

The conditions for public overreaction to unsubstantiated fears were already in place, and there wasn't any time to collect new evidence before silicone hysteria reached an even higher plane. CBS producers for *Face to Face with Connie Chung* were preparing a television exposé that would produce a reaction to breast implants like few other health scares in the nation's history.

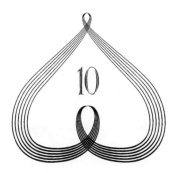

REPORTING THE RUMOR VS. REPORTING THE EVIDENCE

*"The newspaper is a device incapable of discriminating between
a bicycle accident and the collapse of civilization."*
—George Bernard Shaw

*"Journalism is, in fact, no more than gossip carried out
under certain rules."*
—Philip Hilts, *New York Times*[252]

On the evening of December 2, 1990, a popular CBS-TV correspondent opened her weekly television newsmagazine *Face to Face with Connie Chung* this way: "Most of us know little about breast implants. We've seen the ads; we've heard the rumors about which celebrities have them and which don't. But we don't know anything about the dangers." She proceeded to build her case against the device, interviewing along the way Sybil Goldrich and three other women, each telling of horrifying experiences following breast implant surgery. Except for fatigue, which was common to all, their symptoms differed. One described a

flu-like syndrome, a second complained of constant pain throughout her body, and a third reported mouth ulcers, hair loss, and a
rash. Such was the mystery: how to best define the alleged "silicone disease," but nobody involved with this broadcast cared
about precise diagnostic criteria."[253]

On camera experts included Tennessee pathologist Douglas
Shanklin and Canadian chemist Pierre Blais, both of whom were
later disqualified as witnesses in American courtrooms because
of fraudulent qualifications. Yet CBS featured their claims of
illnesses caused by silicone exposure. Without any reference to
four decades of silicone polymer research, Shanklin characterized
the nation's experience with breast implants as an unregulated
experiment that victimized two million unsuspecting women.
He reported evidence of silicone found in the liver and spleen,
omitting the fact that identical findings were recorded for many
without breast implants. Accompanying images were chosen
for their shock value; for example, Blais poking his finger into a
beaker of silicone gel while he spoke of its carcinogenic properties. Omitted entirely was mention of a clinical study showing no
increase in breast cancer among implanted women. Ms. Chung
later boasted: "it was one of the most important stories we've ever
done."[254]

What CBS and the Face to Face team achieved that night was
a new low for one-sided fearmongering journalism. Millions of
viewers, some of them with breast implants and many more with
other silicone exposures, experienced a tsunami wave of terror.
Unlike turn-of-century muckraker Upton Sinclair, who had personally devoted weeks of observation before describing what he
saw, Ms. Chung and her producers had followed the lead of a single consumer activist, Sybil Goldrich, who handpicked the victims
and the corroborating "experts." Chung's report began with an
unproven conclusion: breast implants are untested and therefore
dangerous. The images and copy were assembled to support that
position. It was a proven formula, perfected and popularized by
Don Hewitt, impresario of the hugely successful broadcast phenomenon, 60 Minutes.

Owing to the speed of electronic transmission, the public impact of Connie Chung's broadcast was just as penetrating to the television viewers' psyche as Sinclair's novel had been to its readers a century earlier . . . only faster. The next morning, telephones began ringing in the offices of plastic surgeons nationwide. Women demanded more information about their implants whether or not they were having problems. Appointment registers soon filled. Most plastic surgeons were caught off guard by the assault on their telephone lines and office schedules; not all of them had paid attention to reports of distant FDA hearings where signs of a gathering storm were apparent.[255]

When the results of actual patient surveys conducted by ASPRS were reported in the aftermath of the Connie Chung broadcast, they were largely ignored by the press; any data released by plastic surgery organizations was assumed to be willfully misleading. Sidney Wolfe later exploited the surgeons' data to his advantage. On a television broadcast hosted by Sally Jesse Raphael, he pronounced with mock amusement, "according to the plastic surgeons' own statistics, one in four of those things don't work!" According to his standard, all reports of capsule contraction, however slight, justified implant removal. So much for the view that postop firmness was a side effect instead of a complication.[256]

It wasn't only Sally Jesse Raphael who brought focus to the implant controversy; every afternoon talk show wanted to paint its own portrait of an evolving human tragedy. Television hostess Jenny Jones was eager to reveal her own misadventure with breast implants. Telling her viewers one afternoon that she had grown up, "flat-chested in a Jayne Mansfield era," she announced, "my body just naturally rejects implants." To her national audience, she recalled six operations in eleven years. "I'd sell everything I own to have back the body I gave up." Some viewers wondered why she hadn't just asked for implant removal. Later, her broadcast featured a woman who, in a panic, took a kitchen knife to both breasts and extracted her own implants.[257]

Headlines in the legitimate press were no less sensational than they were in the tabloid press. "One Woman's Case History a Nightmare," was the headline for an article written by Bonnie Winters of the *Kentucky Post*. "FDA accused of downplaying possible breast-implant risk," warned Nancy Benac of The Associated Press. The *New York Times*, long proud of its high standards for science reporting, assigned political reporter Philip Hilts to cover the FDA's maneuvering, and medical reporter, Sandra Blakeslee, to report on the health risks. Her headlines were tabloid in character and calculated to elicit fear. Readers of "Carcinogen found in milk of mom who has implants" were never told that the chemical traces in question had caused tumors only in rats, never humans.[258]

Within a few weeks of *Connie Chung*, the publicity blitz against breast implants had become global in scope. Major network stars, news services, syndicated columnists, and popular magazines all became involved. Whenever this happens in America, a deliberate campaign can often be traced to the skilled efforts of public relations specialists. Fenton Communications, a 1960s creation of David Fenton, is based in the nation's capital and bills itself as America's leading public interest PR firm. In practice, it has produced a long series of remarkably effective fear campaigns, among them the Alar scare with a *60 Minutes* kickoff. In 1990, Fenton began working closely with Sybil Goldrich's network and several trial lawyers. This didn't happen in a PR vacuum however. Dow Corning Corporation contracted for services from Burson-Marsteller and the plastic surgeons signed with Porter Novelli.[259]

The political agendas of advocates such as Sidney Wolfe or a firm such as Fenton are more easily explained than is the motive of a constitutionally protected press deliberately misleading its readers with one-sided reporting. Yet there is a longstanding historical tradition for the press to take sides when reporting a controversy, even a science controversy. Early republic pamphleteers were the forerunners of modern journalism, and they wrote exclusively partisan copy. Not until the mid-nineteenth century and the so-called "penny press" did publications such as James Gordon Bennett's *New York Herald* adopt new objectives: be first with the news, put copies on the street several times a day, appeal to the broadest readership, and do it all for a penny. Newspapers today are accused of abandoning these principles. Opinion is no longer limited to the editorial page. An article's bias is often flagged by its headline. Furthermore, science issues are as politicized as any other subject—consider stem cell research, climate change, genetically modified crops ("frankenfood") to name a few. In 1990, breast implants symbolized big business profiting at the expense of a woman trying to meet male-imposed standards. "This isn't just about breast implants; it's about empowering women," Sybil Goldrich was heard to say.[260]

A smart reporter—one who seeks the editor's approval, plus a banner headline and a byline—learns quickly to focus on journalism's "Four Horsemen of the Apocalypse:" war, famine, death, and disease. Today, the "disease beat" might still involve contagion (as of this writing, it is the Ebola virus), but it can also include a broader array of risks such as trans-fats, high-fructose soft drinks, and of course coffee. Worries about caffeine are as pervasive today as they were throughout Dr. Wiley's government tenure. Because ours is a culture that relishes the kind of news that generates widespread community alarm, editors budget column space or broadcast minutes accordingly. Both print and the broadcast media are sensitive to forces affecting their bottom line, especially in the face of declining circulation.

Print and broadcast news editors commonly feed off of each other's lead stories, resulting in what Brandeis University Professor Susan Moeller calls "compassion fatigue." As director of the journalism program, she points out that incessant coverage of sensational calamities, real or imagined, obscures recognition of authentic problems that people should be doing something about. Mega–media mergers, the tyranny of the bottom line, and a diminishing attention span of the American public aren't helping the problem either.[261]

Health and science reporting doesn't receive the emphasis it deserves in schools of journalism. Newspapers and networks are thus poorly staffed for qualified interpretation of genuine science news. The inevitability of deadlines places limits on a reporter's research time and accuracy falls by the wayside. Collecting an anecdote is as simple as a phone call. Identifying a cohort of alleged victims (the numerator) is moderately challenging. Defining the population from which victims are drawn (the denominator) is extremely difficult and time consuming. And when the editor's assignment involves a lawsuit based on dubious science, the plaintiff attorney's imagined theory of causation is usually more enthralling than the corporation's defense argument. Because the plaintiff's expert witnesses are usually more colorful, they receive more attention than defense experts. By the time research puts to rest a false fear, the press has moved to another health scare, leaving the public in a quandary about what to believe and what to dismiss.

The American Council on Science and Health monitors the media for scientific stories. Nutrition advice is fertile soil for misrepresenting the evidence, it points out, because there are so many bogus organizations claiming professional status (e.g., The American College of Nutripathy) or issuing questionable certificates (e.g., Registry of Colon Therapists). ACSH rates most women's magazines higher for health facts than men's fitness publications. When surveyed, 87 percent of viewers believed they were receiving valid information from the television newsmagazines. But when ninety-seven health-related scripts from 60 Minutes were rated on a scale of 0 (failure) to 4 (excellent), the average grade was 2 (fair). The least reliable segments dealt with Alar (apples), malathion (water supply), and amalgam (dental fillings).[262]

Reporters who insist that they are producing "fair and balanced" reporting can easily mislead their readers when both sides of an issue are given equal weight. Consider the disservice of reporting the latest initiatives of the Flat Earth Society every single time our spherical planet is acknowledged in print. But even if a uniformly high standard of science journalism could be established and maintained, how well prepared is the American public to understand and make use of the information presented? Surveys conducted for the National Science Foundation by Northwestern

University's Center for Biomedical Communications reveal that only 17 percent of Americans were considered science literate in 1999. Fifty-five percent didn't know what DNA meant or why it was important. Only 22 percent could define a molecule, and 55 percent were confused about whether lasers were sound waves or light waves. Featuring the survey's findings on *The Tonight Show,* Jay Leno quipped: "Seventy percent of Americans don't understand science. Thirty percent don't even know what 70 percent means!" But was it a joke or a grim fact?[263]

Statistical interpretation is based on probability that requires an understanding of fractions and decimals. But math teachers admit that probability is no longer taught because statistics problems are word problems and most students entering high school are reading below grade level. Math scores in America are declining and have been for several decades. According to data collected by the Organization for Economic Cooperation and Development (OECD), fifteen-year-olds in the United States rank twenty-fourth among twenty-nine industrialized nations for mathematical skills, just ahead of Portugal and Mexico. Asian nations like Singapore (No. 1), Japan, and Korea stand at the top where US students ranked a generation ago. NYU education historian Diane Ravitch has compared math textbooks over time. In a 1973 algebra textbook, the index listed under F: "factors, factoring, fallacies, finite decimal, finite set, formulas, fractions, and functions." In a 1998 "New Math" text, the index lists under F: "fast food, fat in fast food, Ferris wheel, fish, fishing, flags, flight, floor plan, flower beds, football, and Ford Mustang." Mathematics, she asserts, "is being nudged in a political direction by educators who call themselves 'critical theorists.' "[264]

The impact of student disinterest in high school science and a dumbing down of math requirements show up in our universities. Only the top fifth of our high school students are qualified for advanced study in the sciences, but only half of these will pursue careers in these fields. If only a quarter of our population is science literate in another decade, that leaves three-quarters in the dark about how science affects their lives.[265]

Fortunately, the news about science journalism is not all bad news. Publications exist with a proven record of quality science coverage; they include the *Economist, Christian Science Monitor, Wall Street Journal, New York Times,* and *Chicago Tribune.* But during the months that followed *Connie Chung's* one-sided portrayal of breast implant risk, only a few reporters reported the evidence rather than the rumor.

Elinor Brecher, a feature writer for the *Miami Herald* and an implant recipient herself following double mastectomy, didn't watch the Connie Chung broadcast, but she heard about it and "read it with mounting horror." She also recognized that the message was based on four women's stories and little more of documented value. "It was a warning of what was to come . . . and if all that many women were sick, then where were they?" So she began her study, first by calling her own surgeon and then others: rheumatology organizations, hospitals, etc. It wasn't the way a scientist would have approached the question, yet she came to a conclusion that contradicted what every other journalist was saying. Then she began writing about her findings.[266]

Virginia Postrel, who had previously reported the folly of attributing animal carcinogen risks to the human experience, challenged many of the assumptions made by critics of the breast implant. Believing that Sidney Wolfe's core argument was that breast implants were unnecessary, not that they were unsafe, she asked her readers to consider the implications of allowing political appointees or puritanical pressure groups to determine what was or wasn't necessary for a woman. Based on Sidney Wolfe's criteria, why shouldn't the pill be banned because it wasn't necessary ("Who needs it?")? Everybody could then go back to diaphragms and condoms. Regarding the FDA's exaggerated scrutiny of breast implants, she asked why the female tampon shouldn't also be questioned on the same basis. Like implants, tampons were already in use when regulatory authority was expanded. Like the implant, tampons are "unnecessary" since alternatives exist. Unlike breast implants, she reminded, the tampon had once caused toxic shock syndrome. Hers was surely a different style of argument; regrettably it was hidden in an obscure publication, *Reason*.[267]

John Stossel, coanchor of ABC's *20/20* thinks of himself as a converted consumer reporter who, in addition to winning eighteen Emmy Awards, once earned high praise from Ralph Nader. Stossel tells about his conversion to contrarian skeptic in his autobiographical *Give Me a Break*, a debunking of hucksters and scam artists. In a media environment he characterizes as a "liberal scourge," he denies accusations of a conservative political bias. Instead, he has learned to examine the evidence behind every new scare tactic. Early on, he noticed the prominent role played by trial lawyers. After tracking down questionable testimony from plaintiff experts claiming that immune testing can identify patients with breast implants, Stossel was pleased to report to his viewers that healthy women without breast implants tested positive as well. He takes pride in the fact that "Nader now talks of me like I was afflicted with a mysterious disease."[268]

Gina Kolata, a highly regarded science reporter for the *New York Times* since 1987, was not initially assigned to the breast implant beat but kept her eye on the evidence offered in support of the claimed risks. It simply did not add up for her. "I started to realize that you had to think of plaintiffs' lawyers with the same skepticism as the [implant] companies. I'd always say please send me what you think is the most compelling evidence that leads you to conclude there is a link between these diseases and silicone implants. I got nothing convincing. They just sent me more anecdotal evidence."[269]

Kolata is eminently qualified for her responsibilities. She earned a master's degree in mathematics from the University of Maryland and spent two years at MIT as a doctoral candidate in microbiology. Realizing that she enjoyed writing about science more than participating in its process, she joined *Science* before moving to the *New York Times*. Suspicious of any press release, she prefers to examine the published data directly. "Scientists hide information too . . . not necessarily by intention," she explains, "but rather by organizing the data poorly or omitting answers to important questions." She knows the difference between a case report and an epidemiology report and has the math background to conduct her own statistical analysis.

Like Stossel, Kolata began her coverage of the implant issue by focusing on physician-experts who were cashing in on the controversy. She singled out Dr. Robert Lewy, a Houston internist who, for exorbitant fees, examined women with breast implants, assigned an appropriate diagnosis, forwarded a report to the designated attorney, and waited for his check. For this kind of reporting, Kolata became the target of a blistering campaign to discredit her. Assumed to be the work of Fenton Communications, a report in *The Nation* accused Kolata of being a faithful apologist for corporate science. Her "Sound Science in Journalism" award was demeaned because it came from an organization with corporate support. Nonetheless, her editors urged her to keep on writing.[270]

Meanwhile, Doris Brecher was encountering resistance from her editors at the *Miami Herald*. She had looked into the media prominence of a University of South Florida rheumatologist, Frank Vasey, who had never conducted any research on silicone or breast implants but claimed that a silicone disease existed with as many as ninety symptoms. He became notorious for the ability to diagnose a silicone disorder from behind his desk and recommend implant removal without examining the patient. Brecher recalled, "My editors became uncomfortable with the fact that nobody else was writing the same angle that I was reporting. Then one day they said I was too close to the subject and that was that. I was taken off the implant story and my research came to an end."[271]

Save for the handful of stalwarts who were willing to look past the hype and question the notion of an epidemic of silicone-mediated disorders, the media circus remained on course. Furthermore, it was about to receive a boost from an unexpected confederate in the person of America's most powerful regulator.

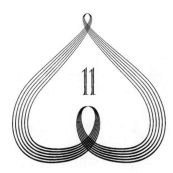

DAVID KESSLER AND
NAKED AMBITION

*"If you had to write a fictional resume for the perfect person to hold
this job, it would turn out to be David Kessler's resume."*
—Peter Barton Hutt, 1991[272]

L ike Harvey Washington Wiley, America's pioneering food
and drug regulator, David Aaron Kessler, MD, JD, was
hailed as one of the best-qualified candidates ever nominated to lead the FDA. In order to secure a position of that
distinction in 1990, appropriate political sponsorship was cru-
cial. Kessler's champion was Utah Republican Senator Orrin G.
Hatch, for whom the doctor had served as a volunteer. Born in
Brooklyn and raised on Long Island in a Republican household,
Kessler's personal inspiration came from a more liberal political
idol: "John Kennedy was president when I was in junior high

school. The message of public service certainly did come across to me."[273]

While his professional education advanced with abundant academic distinction, his aspirations often leaped past one goal to the next. While a liberal arts student at Amherst College, he undertook a study of viral-induced kidney diseases at Sloan-Kettering Institute. While distinguishing himself at Harvard Medical School, he interrupted his progress to study law at the University of Chicago. Acknowledging later that his wife, Paulette, was the real lawyer in the family, he confessed: "I signed up for the courses but only showed up for the exams; law school wasn't that hard. The hardest part was writing the checks." One of his law professors, Richard Epstein, later recalled Kessler: "He was a good student, but not an analytical star by any means. You also knew he wasn't going to spend the rest of his life poking at people's openings."[274]

After receiving his law degree in 1978 and his medical diploma in 1979, Kessler chose Johns Hopkins Hospital for postgraduate training in pediatrics, in part because he would be close to the nation's capital. Needing to justify his decision to specialize in childhood diseases, he said, "When you win, you win big! You win 72 years of life for a person." Yet, he interrupted his clinical training repeatedly with forays to nearby Washington where he pursued his public service ambitions. Later, as FDA commissioner, he would reflect on his attraction to "this town" as he often referred to the capital: "I spent time on the Hill, getting trained, learning how this town works." For the *New York Times,* he compared the relative value of his many steps in training: "I'm supposed to say that my most important training was my medical internship, but frankly, my years on Capitol Hill were the most important. That's what taught me how this town works."[275]

Fellow residents at Hopkins understood that Kessler saw himself as a large-scale manager, a person with enough ambition to get big things done. "If there was a crisis on the floor, David didn't run to the patient; he ran to the phone, calling in the necessary expertise," observed Mark Hudak, another resident at the time. Suddenly faced with responsibility for resuscitating a morbid child in the emergency room, "he ran the code over the phone," eventually assembling the help he required.[276]

Meanwhile, Kessler established a rule with the nurses caring for his patients at night: "Don't take an order from me unless I have both feet on the floor. . . . You'd wake up and you'd find out that you had given an order while you were sleeping." Fellow resident Nancy Hutton recalled an early Saturday morning telephone call: "I'm on the Metroliner. I fell asleep. I'll get there. I'll be on the next [southbound] train." Returning to Baltimore late from Washington and scheduled to assume weekend call duty, an exhausted Kessler with eyes already fixed on high government service had boarded a late evening train, slept through his intended stop, and awakened somewhere in Delaware.[277]

Throughout his residency, Kessler contacted legislators to offer assistance without compensation. Caring little about political party affiliation, he concealed any personal partisan leanings. Neither New York's Republican Senator Jacob Javits nor Massachusetts' Democratic Senator Edward Kennedy had any open positions for him. Eventually, he secured an assignment as staff assistant to Chairman Orrin Hatch's Committee on Labor and Human Resources, the Senate's de facto health affairs committee. At the same time, he was taking MBA classes at NYU and serving as administrative intern at Montefiore Medical Center in the Bronx. In 1982, at the age of 32, he was appointed medical director of the Jack D. Weiler Hospital of the Albert Einstein College of Medicine. Professional colleagues there still remember him as a fair and attentive executive, willing to support the needs of all medical disciplines. Yet he wasn't satisfied with just one major responsibility; Columbia University Law School accepted his offer to teach food and drug law, a field he had never practiced.[278]

Meanwhile, Washington's siren song beckoned political progressives such as Kessler to public service, just as it had tempted Harvey Washington Wiley in 1883. Dr. Kessler was more akin to Wiley in preparation for government service, personal resolve, and temperament than any recent FDA commissioner. Both had avoided shortcuts in their training; both were far more committed to issues than they were to any political ideology. And both were unmistakably driven men. "By the time a person reaches my age, he is supposed to have lost the urgency of ideals . . . but it hasn't worked that way for me," Kessler once said. Asked in 1990 to serve on a Department of Health and Human Services (DHHS) committee to study the apparent ineffectiveness of the FDA, he came under the tutelage of chairman and former commissioner Charles Edwards. What Edwards and fellow committee members saw was an unassuming, sandy-bearded figure with eyeglasses as thick as magnifying lenses and a lightning-fast mind. Later that same year, Dr. Louis Sullivan, DHHS secretary under President George H. W. Bush, summoned Kessler to his office and asked what he would do with the agency. "Enforce the law!" he replied. Sometime later, the secretary's chief of staff, Charles Calhoun, asked Kessler if he planned to be loyal to Sullivan or to his former mentor, Orrin Hatch. The question surprised the nominee because having to be loyal to any individual in Washington had never dominated his thinking about public service.[279]

Throughout his service to the Edwards committee, Kessler knew that the post of FDA commissioner lay empty. When he solicited backing for the post from his burgeoning list of Capital Hill friends, Senator Hatch responded with timely enthusiasm. Because President Bush's aides were troubled by Kessler's apparent lack of party identification, the senior Republican senator's endorsement was essential for the appointment. Additional support from Edwards, who understood what it took to wield a large and complex agency, contributed to one of the fastest congressional confirmations—eight days—in modern history. In November 1990, David A. Kessler, at the age of 39, was sworn in as the youngest commissioner of the Food and Drug Administration since 1912.[280]

Public reaction to the appointment was immediate and flattering. *Time* magazine described Kessler as a man with "endless energy and eagle-scout scruples." *Newsweek* predicted that his "frenetic style will hit the demoralized FDA like electroshock therapy." *People* magazine gushed over his "reputation for incorruptibility." All of these encomiums preceded any significant achievement on Kessler's part. The prestigious and customarily understated journal, *Science,* would only say to its professional readership that the newest FDA commissioner was "an overachiever with all the requisites for his new job." Six months into his term of office, the *New York Times* branded him as the FDA's much-needed "shot in the arm." "After only ten months of service, the *Ladies Home Journal* suddenly announced that Dr. Kessler had already done more to revolutionize the food industry than any federal official in history."[281]

Few doubted that the newest chief executive of one of the most powerful government bureaucracies knew what he was getting into. As every member of the Edwards DHHS committee understood clearly, the FDA was still rebounding from revelations of bribes and kickbacks granted in return for accelerated approvals of generic drug applications. Kessler later recalled, "I came to an agency that had been rocked by scandal and demoralized by the corrupt actions of a few, its resources diminished, its powers of enforcement vitiated. I came to an agency peopled by dedicated professionals who had lost their sense of direction . . . looking for a compass with which to redirect their faith." Months later, when asked whether he had served as the needed compass, he modestly disclaimed his earlier piety: "No, no, this is an agency of wonderful people, 8,000 dedicated public servants. . . . all I had to do was jump-start it."[282]

Scandal and a demoralized staff were the least of his problems. A year before his appointment, a *New York Times* headline read, "A Guardian of Health Buckling under Stress." Because the industries regulated by the FDA were booming, the number of applications for approval of new drugs and devices had risen from 4,200 in 1970 to 12,800 in 1989. Over the same span of years, notifications of serious drug reactions had increased from 12,000 to 70,000. Each year brought another 16,000 reports of problems with medical devices, an increasing number of these involving silicone breast implants. Every year, the agency received 70,000 consumer inquiries and 3,000 queries from members of Congress. And because of the newly enacted Freedom of Information Act (FOIA), the agency was mandated to respond to 40,000 such requests each year, most of them demanding a full accounting of a product's application review. Between 1980 and 1990, Congress had passed twenty-four new laws assigning even more responsibilities to the FDA. Yet under the Reagan administration, regulatory budgets had been reduced. The number of employees working for the agency was down from 7,960 in 1978 to 6,960 in 1987. One-third worked in the field; the rest occupied desks and laboratories in Rockville and Bethesda, Maryland. The law mandated inspection of all food processors at two-year intervals, but eight years might pass without revisits, leaving industry to operate according to an honor system. No surprise that complaints against the FDA for its inefficiency were commonplace.[283]

A call had come from leaders of the pharmaceutical industry to members of Congress demanding that additional financial support be given to the beleaguered agency. A group formed by a melding of professional societies and major companies such as Merck, Johnson & Johnson, Pfizer, and Procter & Gamble were lobbying on behalf of the FDA's interests on Capitol Hill. No one could recall a precedent. Peter Hutt of the firm Covington Burling and former general counsel under Commissioner Edwards remarked, "The FDA's problem is resources . . . a serious erosion across the board. This is the most important regulatory agency in the world; if we harm it, we are taking chances with the public health."[284]

Arriving at FDA headquarters in Rockville, Maryland, soon after his confirmation, Kessler asked the current acting commissioner to stay on and make the key day-to-day decisions while he met with department heads for long-range planning. Unfortunately, crises were the order of the day, and there would be little time for developing strategy. A week hadn't passed when Public Affairs Officer Jeff Nesbit informed the commissioner that cyanide deaths were being reported in the Pacific Northwest because of violated bottles of Sudafed, a nasal decongestant. Kessler's first step was easy: he issued public warnings throughout the Seattle area. More difficult was a decision to force the manufacturer, Burroughs-Welcome, to recall the product, but he did so without hesitation. When a reporter asked why he failed to act even sooner than he did, Kessler began to understand the futility of trying to please everyone.[285]

The commissioner hadn't forgotten his pledge to "enforce the law." He announced his intention to hire one hundred new inspectors trained and experienced in criminal investigation. He talked tough about fairness and honesty in food labeling at his first speech, delivered to an association of attorneys representing industry on food and drug regulatory issues. For anyone with a historical perspective, his language was reminiscent of Dr. Wiley's militant demeanor. Consumer watchdogs had long pushed for a new level of disclosure on food labels, not just the required listing of ingredients but a percentage breakdown, a calculation of caloric value, daily limits for fat grams, sugar, salt, and fiber content. Why, they asked, did Sara Lee "light" cheesecake contain more fat than its regularly labeled version? A new food labeling law, initially resisted by industry because of the confusion it would bring to the marketplace, was passed soon after Kessler settled into his office.[286]

Misuse of the term "fresh" by an industry whose products were processed far from their harvest served as an aggravation to the agency. Kessler didn't need any new laws to enforce dishonest representation of a food product; the 1906 statutory definition of misbranding had been used repeatedly by Dr. Wiley to attack the corn sugar industry, the whiskey rectifiers, and Coca-Cola. Kessler was learning how to draw the maximum public attention to his actions; looking around for his first target, he selected a giant, Procter & Gamble. On April 24, 1991, after company lawyers refused to meet an FDA deadline for correcting the alleged misbranding of their Citrus Hill Fresh Choice Orange Juice, US marshals overran a SuperValu warehouse in Minneapolis and surrounded twenty-four thousand cartons of the product with yellow crime scene tape; technically, it was a government seizure. The event was carefully timed to coincide with a scheduled speech in Florida where Kessler stunned a room full of food executives with an announcement of his action. It was all captured on videotape and within moments played on television screens throughout the nation. Procter & Gamble promptly caved to government pressure, agreed to change its labeling, and donated the "flawed juice" to a local food bank.[287]

Kessler wasn't required to seek approval from his superiors before seizing property as Wiley had been forced to do. In fact, it never occurred to Kessler to notify anyone. Next day, he received a call from Secretary Sullivan's office; an aide advised the commissioner to inform DHHS in advance rather than create a national sensation without letting the boss know first. Undaunted, Kessler proceeded with his truth campaign. He asked why it was not deceptive that dried pastas sitting on grocery shelves at room temperature were labeled "fresh." Then he demanded that Ragu stop claiming its processed spaghetti sauce was a fresh product. In so doing, he unwittingly entered the international regulatory arena where he held no jurisdiction. Ragu was a division of Unilever, the Dutch food giant. Next, Kessler ordered Crisco and Mazola to remove the words "no cholesterol" from their labels. Once again he was stepping beyond his statutory limits; corn oil contains no cholesterol, thereby precluding any valid charge of misbranding. Nonetheless, the commissioner argued that absence of cholesterol in a fat-only product gave false reassurance to consumers seeking a heart-healthy diet. The labeling was quietly changed without argument. He was demonstrating an old principle that power is not only granted but also taken. Meanwhile, staff morale soared at the agency where a banner now spanned the lobby proclaiming, "The watchdog is back and it has teeth." Comedian Jay Leno nominated Bumble Bee Brand Tuna for Kessler's next attack because no bumblebees emerged from a recently opened can. Informed of his media exposure, the commissioner beamed: "I knew the FDA had hit the big time when Leno mentioned us in his monologue."[288]

Kessler was not afraid to take on big issues, and he would eventually challenge "Big Tobacco," arguably the greatest threat to personal health in the nation. For the time being, however, he wasn't grappling with the kind of problems that the FDA needed fixed most quickly. Food company executives complained that the agency was so caught in the glare of klieg lights that it was neglecting its duty to notify industry in advance of compliance deadlines. The commissioner had indeed become a popular subject for network and local news reporters, as well as for the weekly magazines. *People* dubbed him America's "Doctor, Lawyer, and FDA Chief," even featuring the commissioner's six-year-old son, who produced a cartoon showing his dad in a wrestling ring as Hulk Hogan battling a giant container of orange juice labeled "FRESH." But a doubting *Washington Times* editorialist observed, "It's nice to know the FDA has found something to do besides preventing AIDS patients from taking drugs the agency isn't convinced are effective." Malcolm Gladwell, writing then for the *Washington Post*, commented to Jeff Nesbit, "Wake me up when he really does something."[289]

Kessler's own mentors, among them Senator Hatch and former FDA Commissioner Charles Edwards, were critical of a series of insignificant regulatory seizures. Kessler seemed more interested in issues that would guarantee him sufficient publicity. These concerns surfaced again when the agency decided to assail the bottled water industry for misuse of the word "natural." Product seizures might have been significant in Wiley's day, but during Kessler's tenure, they were rarely more than laughable events. Growing suspicions of a self-aggrandizing FDA commissioner were reinforced by news of the next looming controversy: the safety of silicone breast implants. Once again, Kessler appeared to be choosing an issue that would appeal to the press and galvanize public attention to his agency. The resulting storm would first distract, then consume, and eventually handicap an already overwhelmed FDA.[290]

A decision to examine recent claims of silicone biotoxicity preceded Dr. Kessler's confirmation by several months. Acting director of the FDA's Center for Devices and Radiologic Health (CDRH) Walter Gundaker had scheduled a Conference on Silicone in

Medical Devices for February 1991 and invited several dozen participants, most of them scientists and clinicians representing different opinions about the emerging controversy. For two full days, empty seats were a rare commodity in the grand ballroom of Baltimore's Marriott Inner Harbor Hotel. As quickly as chairs were unfolded at the rear of the hall, they were occupied. Conspicuous among the invited participants was a boisterous crowd of consumer advocates, most of them outspoken critics of breast implants. FDA staff organizers managing the meeting reprimanded them frequently for disturbing the proceedings. Less noticeable were print journalists covering the event, and least conspicuous were the attorneys representing plaintiff legal firms, who said little except to each other. They listened and took copious notes.[291]

Although presentations from FDA scientists were muted in tone, the agency's bias against silicone was soon apparent. Dr. Nirmal Mishra spoke once again, as if on cue, about carcinogenic properties for silica and asbestos as if these were chemically related to silicone polymers. Most professionals in the audience understood they were not. Apparently unaware of the position taken by former FDA Commissioner Young regarding the insignificance of animal carcinogen studies, Mishra dwelled on the role of silicone polymers as animal carcinogens, rejecting once again any relevance of clinical data. He was followed by Dennis Deapen, who offered updated findings from the LA/USC epidemiologic study. Women with implants followed now for fifteen years still showed fewer breast cancers than expected for a matched population without the devices.[292]

One panel discussion considered the risk of connective tissue diseases. More case reports were cited; Weisman's recent analysis was brushed aside. Reports of assays implying immune dysfunction were heard, but their significance went unexplained. Hand surgeon Alfred Swanson described a remarkable clinical success with arthritic women, four thousand treated with flexible silicone finger joints. He could not recall a single patient whose arthritic symptoms worsened; x-rays of joints adjacent to the devices showed obvious improvement.[293]

Prior to adjournment, Robert Sheridan of the FDA's Office of Device Evaluation outlined a timetable for the agency's examination of breast implants. Acknowledging that issuance of the final classification in 1988 was four years late, he excused the delay by telling just how busy the agency had been: 3,000 new device applications reviewed, 15,000 investigational device exemptions published, 32,000 premarket notification applications examined, and 910 new regulations written, the latter item bringing groans from the audience. He acknowledged that the FDA could not demand review of any device without just cause, but the request for comments had attracted 2,670 complaints, unprecedented in the agency's history. His best estimate for an application deadline was June 1, 1991 (later revised to July 9, 1991). Nobody was pleased by the news. Surgeons and manufacturers present recognized only the inevitability of looming regulatory power; Sidney Wolfe and fellow critics saw a continuing maize of regulatory obfuscation designed to promote the interests of industry.

On March 25, 1991, Commissioner Kessler took the occasion of Food and Drug Law Institute meeting in Chicago to outline several new enforcement initiatives: more clinical audits, more random inspections, and expanded criminal skills for investigators. Although there was no mention of small arms training, when physician's offices were later raided for medical records, office staff took note that FDA inspectors were armed. Dr. Kessler was fulfilling his promise to enforce the law with all the power he could summon.

Next on the FDA's agenda was the problematic polyurethane-coated implant, a device originally conceived in 1970 by Los Angeles plastic surgeon Frank Ashley. His goal was to eliminate capsule contraction by eliminating the silicone shell's contact with surrounding tissue. Marketed as the Natural-Y or Meme implant depending on who made it, the device drew praise from surgeons who reported softer breasts after replacing the Cronin device with Ashley's product. But there were lingering concerns about the loosely bound coating, among them its metabolic fate. In Canada, where the Delaney Amendment didn't apply, the device was declared safe based on clinical data. In the United States, laboratory analysis revealed trace amounts of 2,4-toluene-diamine (TDA). It didn't take long for implant critics to find a study of rats fed superhuman doses of TDA until tumors appeared.[294]

The Canadian position on polyurethane meant nothing to the FDA. The *New York Times* obliged the agency with a report that seven hundred and fifty thousand women with polyurethane breast implants might be at risk for cancer of the liver. A gross overestimate for sure, and no explanation that laboratory rats are well known for their tumor susceptibility. Suspecting the story's origin, ASPRS challenged the FDA to reveal its evidence for risks considered worthy of press attention.[295]

Answering for the FDA, Dr. Robert Sheridan acknowledged that the press release was unauthorized and promised an internal criminal investigation, a dodge that fooled no one. Nonetheless, the agency's assault on polyurethane continued with an unsubstantiated worst-case lifetime liver cancer risk ratio of 1 in 10,000 women (later reduced to 1 in 1,000,000). There was no good reason to focus on liver cancer, a malignancy known to be decreasing in frequency despite a documented association with viral exposures. All manner of reason had vacated the evaluation of polyurethane as a biomaterial. Meanwhile, Sandra Blakeslee of the *New York Times* added new fuel to the fire: "A cancer-causing chemical has been found in the milk of a nursing mother who had breast implants covered with polyurethane foam." The implication was clear; breast implanted mothers were imparting a cancer risk to their offspring, born and unborn. These were events that foreshadowed the approach regulators would soon take when silicone gel devices came under scrutiny.[296]

The July 31, 1991, meeting of the General and Plastic Surgery Advisory Panel in Gaithersburg, Maryland, was devoted entirely to the polyurethane question. Coated breast implants had achieved sudden notoriety in March of that year when a New York City jury awarded $4.45 million to plaintiff Anna Livshits, a recipient of the device before developing ovarian cancer. Plaintiff attorney Denise Dunleavy had featured Marc Lappe, who as her "expert chemist," convinced the jury that TDA had surely contributed to the plaintiff's course of illness.[297]

At the panel meeting, a battle of the scientists ensued, the FDA's finest versus industry's best. Disagreements over laboratory methods were spirited but most testimony went over the heads of an audience dominated by consumer activists. The damage was already done. FDA officials had previously made clear that they would keep raising the bar until no manufacturer was willing to continue the fight for polyurethane-coated breast implants. Bristol Myers Squibb announced on July 9, 1991, it would remove its product, all because of one animal carcinogen study of dubious clinical relevance, a wildly imaginative cancer risk estimate, and the Delaney Amendment. Meanwhile, the use of polyurethane in other devices such as cardiac pacemakers was never restricted, and its acceptability for breast implants remained valid in Canada and Europe.[298]

In full command of his agency by early summer of 1991, David Kessler was kept informed as deliberations on breast implants evolved. On *Face to Face with Connie Chung,* the FDA was accused of allowing faulty products to be sold to unsuspecting women. Chairman Ted Weiss of the Human Resources Subcommittee promptly scheduled hearings. Kessler immediately announced there would be no more delays or extensions; the review would proceed at once.

Four manufacturers met the July 9, 1991, deadline. Dow Corning's subsidiary responsible for manufacturing and distributing plastic surgery products, Dow Corning Wright (DCW) submitted two PMAs, one for single lumen and the other for double lumen implants. Each application amounted to fifty-seven volumes, encompassing more than thirty years of manufacturing processes, product design, labeling, safety studies, warnings, and market surveillance. Because the FDA stipulated that five copies be submitted using two-inch binders, this meant 570 volumes of data shipped from DCW's Arlington, Tennessee, facility. Supplements, updates, and amendments would later add to that number.

Mentor Corporation submitted three PMAs, Inamed (formerly McGhan), Medical Engineering Corp/Surgitek, Bioplasty, and Cavon Corporation had one each for a grand total of nine. Because these manufacturers could not cite research as far back as the 1940s, their applications were less imposing, but it all represented a daunting burden (more than one million pages according to estimates) for an overwhelmed agency expected to review the information in time for the next advisory panel meeting, November 12–14, 1991.[299]

But Kessler needed something more visibly decisive for Congress than an application deadline. Inspectors soon found him the opportunity he sought, in a warehouse outside of St. Paul, Minnesota. Although Bioplasty had met the recent PMA deadline for silicone gel implants, it had also filed an IDE for a novel breast implant with an alternative filler trademarked as "bio-oncotic gel." Biologically inert and efficiently excreted by the kidney without physiologic residuals, its golden color prompted the device's trade name, MISTI-Gold. The FDA had given its approval for clinical trials only, stipulating that the product must not be marketed as an agency-approved device. Bioplasty erroneously assumed the agency would not make a distinction between its novel device and silicone gel devices currently under review. It was an error Kessler chose to exploit, thereby demonstrating to Congressman Weiss that the FDA was serious about regulating the breast implant.[300]

Tipped off in advance by the FDA, television news teams filmed the seizure, and major networks jumped onto the story for their evening broadcasts. Five hundred pairs of implant shells were taken, along with another five hundred packages of the organic gel used to fill them. It was the beginning of the end for Bioplasty as a device manufacturer. Their pleas and reminders that the MISTI device had been approved for trial use went unheeded. The FDA in August rejected the IDE application filed the month before. Foreign sales weren't sufficient to sustain the company. In time, bankruptcy would be the only practical choice.

Near the end of summer, ASPRS President Norman Cole met with his board of directors to review the outcome of July's events; two clinically effective products were now removed from the market in response to FDA pressure. Curious about Dow Corning Wright's reaction to these events, he consulted Director of Marketing Gene Jakubczak. Were all breast implants now at risk he asked? Cole later recalled being told it was a manufacturer's problem. Plastic surgeons had nothing to worry about, according to Jakubczak, who boasted of the twenty-two-foot-high stacks of bound volumes recently shipped. But Cole had serious concerns about the company's ability to convince the FDA of anything. When he subsequently learned the FDA was critical of manufacturers for not offering proof that the devices actually did enlarge a woman's breast contour, it was apparent that "an organized effort to torpedo the breast implant was underway."[301]

Cole's doubts might have been amplified had he been present on a September morning when Dow Corning Wright's Bob Rylee took a call from *New York Times* reporter Philip Hilts asking for reaction to the FDA's listing of deficiencies in the company's two breast implant applications. Rylee had not received his copies, but they were already in the hands of the press; they could only have come to them from the FDA. The two eight-page documents enumerated both minor and major deficiencies and offered the company an opportunity to file amendments to their applications. But that would be taken by the FDA as application withdrawal, thereby starting the clock all over again. Upon the advice of its lawyers, DCW chose to address deficiencies at the next panel meeting rather than suffer the consequences of a withdrawn application. It had two months to prepare better explanations of the data, perhaps update the evidence. The mood was no longer optimistic. Some recall "the day of deficiencies" had come on Friday the thirteenth.[302]

Girding for what it assumed would become a pitched battle with government, the ASPRS board of directors met to consider a special assessment of its members. Seven hundred and fifty thousand dollars had been raised to confront the FTC in 1977. If organized plastic surgeons were going to wage battle with the FDA successfully, they would need a larger war chest. Not all members believed that pugnacity in the face of regulatory power was a wise stand for a professional organization, but the resolution passed easily. Members were asked to pay $350 annually over the course of three years, and nearly every surgeon complied. Out of $3.1 million collected, $500,000 was allocated for additional silicone device research to be conducted independent of the device manufacturers. The remainder would be used for public education and outreach, including costs of public relations consultants believed necessary to put the surgeons' case before the public.[303]

As the November hearings approached, ASPRS could anticipate the coming media circus and a particularly bad wave of publicity. And so its consultants conceived a "patient fly-in." Women willing to speak publicly about their satisfaction following breast surgery would come to the nation's capital to voice a contrasting message. With an assist from Burson-Marsteller, the press was alerted to the arrival of nearly six hundred women and plastic surgeons. For three days in October 1991, they visited their respective legislators and demanded the right of women to choose implants if they wished. Clever perhaps (a few thought it bizarre), but it backfired even before the drama played to its final curtain. For every satisfied patient, Fenton Communications offered two more willing to relate the agony of their silicone ailments. Public Citizen knew which group would attract the most media attention.[304]

Another breast implant spectacle was budding in San Francisco. Mariann Hopkins, who had selected her attorney, Dan Bolton, from a 1988 television news broadcast, was about to have her day in court. Characterized as the scrappy wife of a firefighter, she had received Dow Corning implants in 1976 following a double mastectomy for cystic disease believed precancerous at the time. Three years later, she was placed on high doses of corticosteroids for a relentless form of connective tissue disease. She would always believe it a miracle that she had turned her TV on just in time to hear Sybil Goldrich describe her misery. Bolton had assembled an impressive list of experts on her behalf. Arguing for Dow Corning was Frank Woodside, who put the plaintiff's own physician on the stand to establish that the patient's rheumatic symptoms preceded the implants by several years. Undeterred by the weakness of his medical case, Bolton kept turning to the incriminating documents that won him victory in the Stern case nine years earlier. The trial began early in November, spanned the device panel's November meeting, but wouldn't reach a verdict until December.[305]

On the evening of Nov. 8, just four days before the FDA hearing began, CBS reran its notorious 1991 breast implant episode renamed *Eye to Eye with Connie Chung*, this time with an updated introduction: "We have some very emotional stories for you tonight, including some that will anger you. In fact, our first story inspired a national letter-writing campaign to CBS and over seven thousand letters." Chung offered no breakdown of the content of those responses but did acknowledge that after the first broadcast, CBS heard from a few women who were happy with their breast implants. She also pointed out that the majority of plastic surgeons believe that breast implants are safe. Chung also reiterated that her 1991 story was "one of the most important we've ever done."[306]

Immediately prior to the hearing, panel secretary Paul Tilton announced that Dr. Elizabeth Connell, professor of gynecology and obstetrics at Emory University Medical School, had agreed to chair the panel, replacing Dr. Norman Anderson, who could never hide his disdain for breast implants. Although manufacturers had long protested his panel leadership, he retained his voting membership. Consumer groups objected to participation from plastic surgeons who had shown their bias by contributing to the ASPRS war chest. The FDA agreed, and three previously appointed surgeons were stripped of their voting rights but retained as consultants. Also added as nonvoting consultants were Kathleen Anneken of Command Trust Network, Marc Lappe, and another of Dan Bolton's scheduled experts for the San Francisco trial, Nir Kossovsky.[307]

There was palpable tension in the air on the morning of Tuesday, November 12, 1991, as FDA staff completed their final arrangements while every seat in the grand ballroom of the

Gaithersburg Holiday Inn was taken. Even before dawn, network and cable technicians worked to install broadcast equipment sufficient to replace three back rows of seats with a double bank of cameras. There would be no limit to coverage of the breast implant issue on that day or the next. In the hallways, Sybil Goldrich and her following were already available to reporters. By prior agreement, the advisory panel was off limits to the press until the hearings were adjourned. After voting members and consultants took their places on stage, Commissioner Kessler offered a welcome to all and a charge to the panel: proceed methodically with careful consideration of a device the agency considered problematic. He was not seen again at the hearing.[308]

The first morning was given to public witness testimonials, some for approving the device, many more for demanding a permanent ban on all silicone implants. Did they mean catheters, shunts, wrist joints, and pacemakers as well? The afternoon was devoted to statements from professional organizations, among them the American Cancer Society, the American Medical Association, and the American College of Radiology. All favored approval of the breast implant because disapproval would lead to restrictions on other devices, some of them lifesaving. Dr. Maurice Jurkiewicz, a plastic surgeon himself, spoke on behalf of the American College of Surgeons. He applauded the FDA for its review of the breast implant but cautioned the panel to consider the enormous benefits of silicone for patients seeking reconstruction of a missing breast. He expressed disappointment that the panel's surgeons, more experienced dealing with implant recipients than any other panelist, had been denied their voting rights. The rest of the afternoon was filled with more testimonials, a parade of one horror story after another. A representative of the National Organization of Women (NOW) spoke ill of women who believed they needed implants, contradicting a principle the organization had long stood for: a woman's right to choose. Later challenged, she added, "We do not support a choice to die!"[309]

The next morning Dow Corning presented a summary of its data followed by Mentor, and on the third day, Inamed and

Bioplasty. The agency had previously refused to evaluate data submitted by Surgitek and Cavon. Each corporate presentation led off with its own scientists followed by invited experts. An FDA reviewer critiqued each presentation based only on the data submitted the prior summer. The agency stood firm on the statutory exclusion of data collected since the original submission, eliminating most of Dow Corning's thunder. For example, Dr. Brody was not permitted to provide the panel with the latest update on his epidemiologic study of breast cancer risk following implantation. Although Inamed CEO Jan Varner would receive compliments in private from an FDA staffer for his company's presentation, public praise for any implant manufacturer was a rare commodity, and it was obvious to all that Dow Corning was taking the brunt of the agency's scorn.[310]

Former panel chairman Anderson asked Dow Corning Technical Director Robert Levier to explain what he meant by his company standing behind all of its implants; did he include every device implanted since 1962? By asking that question, Anderson had exceeded PMAA parameters and the audience knew it. But there were no objections heard from any FDA representative.[311]

Chairwoman Connell did her best to mediate a rational inquiry given an emotionally charged audience and so many confounding regulations. Her exhaustion was apparent by the afternoon of the third day, but she forged ahead with a polling of panelists still eligible to vote. It came as no surprise that all applications were rejected because "none provided reasonable assurance that the devices were safe and effective under the conditions of use described." The panel's remaining issue to consider was future product availability despite the deficiencies. Although a few, like Norman Anderson, were steadfast on banning the devices, an easy majority voted to permit "continued availability of silicone gel-filled prostheses because such availability is necessary for the public health." The needs of the breast cancer victim remained important when the panel's choice of language was established.[312]

Before adjournment, nonvoting members were allowed to offer closing statements. Citing twenty-seven years of experience using breast implants without intending harm, plastic surgeon Thomas Krizek objected to his loss of voting privilege. Why, he asked, was the breast implant receiving more attention than the silicone device in his reconstructed wrist? He decried the message soon to be heard by two million women with implants: "These are not FDA approved but don't worry about it." Next up, Marc Lappe, who acknowledged his role in prior litigation but didn't think he was "any less pure than anyone else on the panel."[313]

Back in a San Francisco courtroom, Mariann Hopkins approached the witness stand with the assistance of a cane. Jurors listened raptly as she described the suffering she had endured since her first breast implant operation. Attorney Bolton understood that success depended on proving that Mrs. Hopkins was severely ill, so he encouraged his client to take all the time she needed; her testimony with wavering of voice took a day and a half. For proof that her implants were the cause of her illness, Bolton called on his chosen experts, Frank Vasey, the Florida rheumatologist, and Nir Kossovsky who was fresh from the recent FDA hearing. Kossovsky charmed the jury with a stylized version of silicone's influence on the immune system, not one of his theories supported by valid evidence. Vasey summarized an extensive experience treating breast implant patients with autoimmune manifestations similar to the plaintiff's. The defense emphasized that her symptoms, according to her own physician, had preceded her diagnosis in 1979, her rupture in 1977, her implantation in 1976. But Dr. Vasey's clinical opinion carried the day: "a silicone related disease."[314]

Not yet certain the entire jury was in his camp, Bolton shocked them with evidence of willful corporate fraud. Memoranda revealing that salesmen in the field were advised to wipe a sticky layer off implants before showing them to surgeons was taken to mean that leakage, however subtle, represented a hazard. Bolton featured another sales rep's comment: "with crossed fingers, I offered that research would be conducted that would provide answers." It would be immortalized as the "crossed fingers memo." Even the plaintiff was stunned by what she heard in the courtroom; Bolton had planned for displays of emotion from his client by withholding evidence from her in advance of the trial.

Dow Corning, still confident that the plaintiff's doctor had destroyed the prosecution's causation argument, offered to settle for two hundred thousand dollars, a generous offer it believed. Bolton wasn't interested; nor did his client wish to settle. On December, 13, 1991, the jury returned a unanimous verdict in favor of the plaintiff, awarding eight hundred and forty thousand dollars in compensatory damages. When the judge asked about additional awards, the foreman announced another unanimous decision: $6.5 million in punitive damages! The courtroom erupted and reporters raced to phone their editors. It was strike three for Dow Corning and within a few weeks, the company would be out . . . out of the breast implant business altogether and facing an indemnity risk of several billion dollars. Once again, breast implants captured national headlines: "Dow Corning Suffers $7.3 Million Judgment!"

A mixed message from the advisory panel wasn't the only disturbing news about breast implants that reached Dr. Kessler's desk during the closing weeks of 1991. From San Francisco came a portfolio of damning memoranda omitted from Dow Corning's recent PMAA. *San Francisco Chronicle* reporter Seth Rosenfeld, who had covered the Hopkins trial, came into possession of the entire document set, forwarded it to Norman Anderson, who in turn transmitted everything to Kessler. In a cover letter, Anderson listed the specific memos he believed the commissioner should examine without delay, then urged a full investigation to learn why Dow Corning had not been forthcoming with the agency. Anderson went on to excoriate Kessler and the FDA for its conduct of the recent hearing, believing that if more panel members had been informed of implant failures, the product would not remain in continued patient use.[315]

Dow Corning Wright's president and CEO, Dan Hayes, realized there was no hope of maintaining the desired court-imposed seal on the San Francisco trial evidence. The whole world seemed to know of the contents. Sidney Wolfe, who had his own set of what came to be known as "Ninety-Nine Dow Corning Documents," forwarded Dr. Anderson's damning letter to Philip Hilts at the *New York Times,* whose account appeared on December 21. When Congressman Weiss received copies for study, he asked the Department of Justice to conduct a criminal investigation of Dow Corning. Unable to stay ahead of the avalanche of damning news, Hayes wrote Kessler: "One of the most disturbing allegations Dr. Anderson makes in his letter is that we are withholding data or studies from the agency. This assertion is unfounded and incorrect. Dow Corning has fully responded under the PMA regulations."[316]

At first reference to the existence of withheld documents, ASPRS requested and received copies by express return mail. Neither Dow Corning nor any other implant maker had ever denied plastic surgeons information they requested. Careful study of the so-called "Ninety-Nine Docs" revealed nothing of clinical significance that the surgeons hadn't already seen and evaluated, surely no new hidden clinical risks. Consumer advocates had already assembled a massive list of implant risks beyond the collective imaginations of manufacturers and surgeons alike. All that was known about gel bleed had been determined in university laboratories with industry support. More definitive answers to the cancer and connective tissue questions would come only from established protocols and the passage of time. But this was not how the commissioner viewed the problem. He now held the evidence that produced the Hopkins verdict. What would he do with it?

Kessler had learned during his fresh orange juice crusade never to blindside a department head, so he remembered to keep DHHS Secretary Sullivan informed about the breast implant dilemma the agency faced. When asked later about those briefings, Sullivan recalled how conflicting the evidence appeared to be at the time. Unlike Kessler, he had practiced medicine for many years before his cabinet appointment and could understand the patient's perspective. He asked Kessler for enough flexibility in the restrictions to assure that women seeking breast reconstruction following mastectomy would have full access to the devices. His

Before	*After*

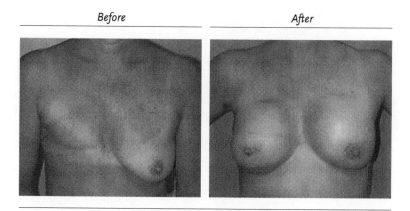

46 yr. old professor following right mastectomy for an advanced breast cancer; delayed reconstruction using tissue expander followed by implant. Mastopexy and implant on left for symmetry. CREDIT: Anne Wallace MD

plea echoed those coming from a majority of the advisory panel. Beyond that, the decision was the commissioner's to make.[317]

Fully qualified in medicine and the law, David Kessler knew something about legal evidence, how it was selectively assembled, and how it could be abused. He had never practiced law, but he was familiar with the tactics used by litigators to vanquish opponents in the courtroom. He was also well versed in the methods that science requires. As a college student he had conducted experiments under close supervision at the Sloan-Kettering Institute. In residency he learned to weigh the medical evidence supporting alternate treatment regimens. For the implant decision he faced, the law offered him circumstantial evidence of a kind that abounds at trials. Science, on the other hand, offered him only absence of proof of disease causation. Now he had to decide which kind of evidence was more useful for defending the statutes his agency was required to enforce and for satisfying his own personal ambitions.

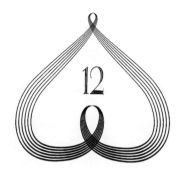

A "MORATORIUM"
AND ITS FALLOUT

"We know more about tires and how long they last than we know about breast implants."
—David Kessler[318]

"How scientific is the FDA's decision that no woman should have implants put in, and no woman should have them removed?"
—Congresswoman Marilyn Lloyd[319]

A press conference scheduled for January 6, 1992, to announce the appointment of Jane Haney as Deputy Commissioner allowed David Kessler an opportunity to resolve what must have been foremost on his mind for several weeks. Mentioning briefly Dr. Haney's distinguished career as a National Cancer Institute scientist, he abruptly changed topics. "Today, I am requesting a moratorium on the further use of all silicone gel breast implants until our advisory committee panel of experts can reconvene to consider new information bearing on the safety of these devices. We want surgeons to stop using these implants in patients until this new information can be thoroughly evaluated." He did not explain what the new evidence was that warranted such an action. When asked by a reporter whether his decision had been influenced by recent litigation, Kessler acknowledged he was aware of recent court actions and the agency was committed to examining every report of serious illness affecting women with breast implants. He emphasized that the FDA was not urging women with breast implants to go have them removed. An agency spokesman later suggested that the risk of removing implants might exceed the risk of leaving them in place, a position plastic surgeons took particular note of because they knew very well that the risk of removing breast implants was slight.[320]

Caveat emptor had never served as a principle the FDA based its policies upon—not under Dr. Wiley a century before and certainly not under Dr. Kessler. And so a decision was announced that would reverberate globally like no regulatory decision ever before. His unprecedented action is remembered as the FDA's breast implant ban, but in reality, it was a plea for surgeons to voluntarily cease using silicone gel breast implants until the agency could review what it believed was new and alarming evidence, information that came from a courtroom rather than from any clinic or laboratory. The FDA held no enforcement authority over the medical profession, and Congress was not likely to grant that power even on an ad hoc basis. The agency also informed manufacturers that all distributed product, including implants held in consignment, were to be recalled without further delay.

The public's reaction was immediate, and it ranged from euphoria on the part of activists like Sybil Goldrich to generalized anxiety for several hundred thousand women with implants already in place. Goldrich characterized the moratorium as a major triumph, and Sidney Wolfe declared Kessler's action a partial victory. ASPRS President Cole challenged Kessler to honor his Hippocratic oath . . . to do no harm. Dr. Cole spoke for ASPRS and his colleagues when he pointed out that plastic surgeons were placed in an untenable position: unable to counsel their patients because the agency had not revealed the "new evidence" leading to its decision. Cole demanded an immediate and full disclosure of any implant risk data held by the agency. But the commissioner didn't have any more evidence than the surgeons were already aware of. All he had were the so-called "smoking gun" memoranda culled from Dow Corning's files by Dan Burton, none of it containing proof of a link between silicone polymers and any cancer, any connective tissue disease, or any other medical infirmity.[321]

As for the many women with breast implants, learning that a powerful and respected federal agency believed that something was seriously wrong with silicone devices sent many of them over the edge emotionally. Not helping were the print reporters who offered readers the gloomiest outlook and exaggerated lifetime hazards. Broadcast media embellished the risks with lurid graphics showing dissemination of silicone, like a giant inkblot spreading from the breast region to the fingers and toes. These images were based entirely on the imagination of artists, not from confirmed evidence of fractions of an ounce of total silicone migration.

Commissioner Kessler made himself immediately available to the media and especially to selected broadcast appearances. On the January 8, 1992, *Diane Rehm Show*, he justified his decision by saying that there was "no data . . . simply no data after thirty years on the market," a falsehood that would have confounded industry executives who had dispatched several hundred boxes of data to FDA headquarters. Immediately recanting, he admitted to receiving "a lot of data but none of it was acceptable." He failed to tell his national audience that the devices had met every accepted standard of the American Society of Testing Materials (ASTM). When asked about the risk of autoimmune disease, Kessler acknowledged that no proof of a causal link existed and estimated that very few women would be found susceptible to silicone reactions. This was just two days after calling for the moratorium, so what was his basis for the action? How appropriate was it for a regulator to depend on speculation for an unprecedented device restriction? Answers were not forthcoming.[322]

Editorial writers for the major newspapers took positions consistent with their publication's established political leaning.

"Wise Timeout on Breast Implants" declared the *New York Times*: "Science Abdicates" countered the *Wall Street Journal*. Declaring the FDA's action a victory for the contingency-fee lawyers, the journal accused "David Kessler JD MD" of "suspending the apparatus of science and invoking the tactics of the courtroom." Writing in *Forbes*, Manhattan Institute fellow Peter Huber asked why there weren't cries of outrage from the advocates of women's choice in matters of intense privacy such as breast surgery? But the ACLU and other prochoice organizations were largely silent on this issue. Not so the Washington Legal Foundation, blasting the FDA for exceeding its statutory authority and retaining consultants who had received payments for implant trial testimony.[323]

Telephones rang incessantly in plastic surgeons' offices throughout the nation. No longer did it matter that patient surveys had shown 95 percent or greater satisfaction rates following breast enlargement surgery. Nearly every caller, most without medical complaints of their own, asked pointed questions in their quest for reassurance. What about these horrific reports on television and in the daily newspapers, many asked. The prudent surgeon made available all the time needed to explain everything known and what was not yet understood about disease relationships. A spot telephone survey of more than three hundred members conducted by ASPRS showed that many patients were asking for removal of their implants regardless of the nature of the evidence yet to be revealed. By the end of 1992, the profile of breast surgeries performed by plastic surgeons had changed entirely: fewer augmentations, more implants removed, breast lifts completed without use of an implant. Regrettably, there were fewer postmastectomy breast reconstructions even though saline-filled implants were available without restrictions.[324]

Norman Cole wrote Dr. Kessler again on April 17: "I am appalled to learn that you do not plan to include women facing mastectomies . . . and wanting immediate reconstruction . . . in the "urgent need" category for use of gel-filled implants." Having previously indicated he would allow access to the gel devices through an adjunct protocol, his April 21 reply omitted any concern for

patients currently in the process of treatment. Instead he reminded Dr. Cole of the obvious; namely, that saline-filled implants were
still available. Then, as a nonpracticing pediatrician, he proceeded
to counsel Dr. Cole about the advantages of breast-preserving surgery for the cancer patient.[325]

Dow Corning Wright employees wondered whether news
favorable to the company would ever come their way again. First,
they had endured the foreboding deficiency letters, followed by the
advisory committee's disapproval of the PMAs, then the Mariann
Hopkins verdict, and finally the unthinkable, a moratorium on
the sale of new product, something nobody in Midland had even
imagined. As had occurred in the 1940s, Dow Chemical was consulted for help, and it came in the person of Keith McKennon, who
had learned his lessons in crisis management while negotiating a
one hundred eighty million dollar settlement of two hundred and
fifty thousand claims against Dow for alleged toxicity from wartime use of the defoliant, Agent Orange. On medical leave at the
time of the moratorium, McKennon agreed to take charge immediately. One of his earliest decisions was to take the company out
of the breast implant business altogether and in time cease production of plastic surgery implants and related products, much to
the dismay of employees who regarded the move an admission
of guilt. He would later explain that the Dow Corning trademark
was unlikely to fare well in the marketplace anytime soon if ever
again. Dow Corning was fated to become again what it had been
at the time of its creation, a source supplier of silicone polymers,
but later resumed its role as a health products innovator minus its
plastic surgery product line.[326]

McKennon urged Vice President and Manager of Corporate
Communications Barie Carmichael to maintain an open posture
with the public, while at the same time courting the press and
acknowledging the company's understanding of the fear experienced by thousands of women. McKennon brought from Dow
Chemical a talented epidemiologist, Ralph Cook, to sort the evidence available, good and bad, and mastermind the conduct of
additional studies. Dow Corning owed its customers answers to

many questions. McKennon, like Coca-Cola's Asa Candler, found himself in an entirely defensive position, yet he prepared to invest whatever resources were required for the research needed to achieve success in the courtroom.[327]

Regulatory bureaus in foreign nations such as France, Italy, and Germany responded indifferently to the breast implant scare. Their habit was to defer to their professional organizations. In Australia, where the government was in the habit of financing consumer groups and relying on their recommendations for policy decisions, a polarization of medical professionals, activists, and solicitors soon reached incendiary level. Not so In the United Kingdom, where the Medical Devices Directorate wasted no time assembling its own expert advisory group to review the existing evidence. Efforts to communicate with the FDA failed to yield even the courtesy of a letter in response. By April 1992, barely three months after the Kessler announcement, the British panel concluded that "there was no evidence of increased risk of connective tissue disease in patients who had undergone silicone gel breast implantation and there was no scientific case for changing policy in the UK with respect to breast implant surgery." All physicians and surgeons practicing in the UK were so informed by the Department of Health's Chief Medical Officer, Kenneth Kalnan.[328]

Back at FDA headquarters, staff wasted no time preparing for the extra panel hearing the commissioner stipulated within forty-five days of the declared moratorium. On February 18, 1992, a revised advisory panel assembled at the Bethesda Marriott Hotel for three more days of deliberations. In response to Inamed suing the agency for slipshod management of the previous hearing, changes were made in the status of Norman Anderson, Marc Lappe, and Nir Kossovsky, each one losing their voting privilege but remaining as consultants. Reacting to criticism that the field of rheumatology was not represented, the FDA invited two professors of medicine as consultants, John Sergent of Vanderbilt University, president of the American College of Rheumatology; and Nathaniel Zvaifler of UC–San Diego, editor of the journal *Arthritis and Rheumatism*.

This time, knowing that he had unleashed a wild bull, Kessler arranged his schedule so he could be present to hear the so-called new evidence along with everybody else. Yet, instead of leading off with autoimmune disease, the issue that elicited the record-breaking punitive damage award, the agency devoted its first morning session to a discussion of device failure and reoperation rates. Two radiologists presented mammograms and ultrasound scans showing suspected but unconfirmed rupture rates in the range of 5 to 11 percent, far higher than any plastic surgeon had ever encountered in practice. Quick to spot inherent bias in the study model, new panel member and Professor of Radiology James Potchen cautioned everyone to withhold judgment. All subjects were women specifically referred for imaging studies because of signs suggesting implant rupture. Short of implant removal, only magnetic resonance imaging, a costly technology, was capable of actually finding a rupture. Furthermore, asymptomatic women are unlikely to pursue diagnostic studies at their own expense. These caveats notwithstanding, the calculated emotional impact of the agency-sponsored reports was achieved; the press reported that 15 percent of all implanted breast devices might already be ruptured.[329]

The afternoon session was taken up with case reports of scleroderma and other rheumatic diseases appearing in women following breast enlargement. Ostensible victims were helped to the microphone nearest to them, some with crutches, others in wheelchairs, a few equipped with nasal oxygen. Dr. Kessler's specially appointed rheumatologic consultants listened attentively to each presentation and then offered their opinions. Dr. Zvaifler pointed out that the relative frequency of the various autoimmune diseases is well known and because so few women with breast implants had developed the most common of them, rheumatoid arthritis, if he were to go on the basis of reports heard that day, he would have to conclude that silicone devices protected patients from developing rheumatoid arthritis. Far better, he added, to conclude that the patient sample was heavily biased. Dr. Sergent observed that the predominant clinical evidence offered that day came from physicians who accepted a link between breast implants and rheumatic disease, thereby influencing which patients came to them for a confirmed diagnosis. Most were, in fact, receiving their referrals from advocacy groups and trial attorneys. Neither consultant believed anyone was taking seriously the probability of coincidental occurrence, an explanation first offered by UCSD rheumatologist Michael Weisman.

On the morning of the second day, device manufacturers were allowed to rebut attacks heard ever since the previous hearing. But first, Tennessee Congresswoman Marilyn Lloyd was afforded the courtesy of opening that session. A breast cancer victim herself, she never took her eyes off Commissioner Kessler when she asked, "How scientific is the FDA's conclusion that no woman should have implants put in, and yet no woman should have them removed?" Revealing that her own course of breast reconstruction had been interrupted by the moratorium, she added, "Silicone gel implants were to be my choice, and they marked the final stage in my recovery from breast cancer, restoring the disfigurement of my surgery." She reminded the commissioner that his arbitrary action had denied her a choice made in collaboration with her surgeon, who unlike Kessler was a practicing professional. Reflecting on the dreadful message transmitted by the agency to several hundred thousand women at a moment when no proof of cancer or autoimmune disease risk was established, Lloyd accused the commissioner of self-serving motives, adding that "It is absolutely not in the realm of this panel or the FDA to determine the political correctness of women who seek implants."[330]

Silence followed her dramatic statement but not for long. Soon women lined up at microphones to offer praise for Dr. Kessler's demonstration of courage and plead for an end to breast implants for any reason, including cancer. One woman used baldness for analogy: if men can adapt to loss of hair, they can adapt to a woman losing a breast without having to expose herself to a toxic substance. Not one of the afternoon critics appeared the least reassured by opinions from the FDA's chosen rheumatology consultants.

The third and final day was set aside for panel deliberations. Dr. Connell, who had waged a continuous battle to maintain order throughout the hearing, now had to persuade members to reach constructive conclusions. Unchanged from the prior hearing was agreement that manufacturers had not yet documented the safety of their product. Nonetheless, the panel urged continued implant availability but with restrictions: "there should be granted a limited access to breast implants and that these limitations should be in terms of carefully controlled protocols." Neither the language nor intent was clear, but it was sufficient for the FDA to later establish a confounding set of regulations.

Testifying months later before the U. S. House of Representatives Subcommittee on Human Resources, Dr. Connell glossed over the continuous acrimony displayed at both hearings. Instead, she emphasized the good that came from those deliberations, among them the panel's belief that the devices met a public need and should continue to be available. Also present was Dr. Sergent who bluntly declared, "the panel was uniquely unqualified for determining such problems as these [rheumatic disease causation]." He went on to question the potential for conducting valid epidemiologic studies given a legally charged environment where monetary incentives elicit subjective symptoms unrelated to any authentic disease process.[331]

Disparagement of a seriously flawed review made little impact on Dr. Kessler. On April 16, 1992, he announced a lifting of the moratorium yet continued to restrict access by imposing requirements for "acquiring once and for all the information necessary to establish the safety of these devices." In other words, silicone gel implants would be available only after manufacturers met protocol standards not yet defined by the FDA, a task the agency had little experience with. He disagreed with the idea that devices have to be proved unsafe before the FDA can act. The law, he noted, places the burden on manufacturers to prove the safety of a device. But until the agency produced its protocol for this research, women seeking either breast reconstruction or cosmetic enlargement were functionally limited to the saline-filled devices.

Congresswoman Lloyd was not the only member of Congress to question Dr. Kessler's moves. A deliberative body populated by 234 lawyers ought to have recognized what was going on. In a letter signed by Tennessee Senator Albert Gore and nine other representatives of his state, the commissioner was urged to balance the adverse evidence with the favorable breast implant experience of many thousands of women over the course of several decades. Twenty-eight members of Congress signed a letter appealing directly to Secretary Sullivan, pointing out that categorizing the breast implant as an investigational device meant loss of insurance reimbursement for mastectomy victims seeking breast reconstruction. Many hundreds of women were, in fact, refused payment for the costs of their reconstructive surgery when insurance companies, looking for a reason not to pay, cited the newly designated investigational status of the device. Yet women seeking removal of their implants were rarely denied reimbursement. Explantation was now considered a medically indicated procedure.[332]

Commissioner Kessler received an unexpected rebuke from Dr. Marcia Angell, associate editor of the highly respected *New England Journal of Medicine*. She wasn't buying any of his arguments. Under the title, "Breast Implants: Protection or Paternalism," she reminded the commissioner that every device carries some risk, that the agency's mandate does not include avoidance of all untoward effects. Responding to the agency's position that any benefits are only cosmetic, she asked, "What does that have to do with anything? Given the challenge of defining subjective benefits, the FDA acted as if there were no benefits." Angell also objected to coercing women into becoming subjects of clinical research protocols. This, she added, was a clear violation of federal regulations guaranteeing that participation in human research must be entirely voluntary. She decried the agency-prompted fears of a million women being "out of all possible proportion to what is known about the risks." She said, "Targeting a device used only by women raises the specter of sexism—either in permitting the use of implants in the first place or in withdrawing them." She reminded Kessler that "people are regularly permitted to take risks much greater than the probable risk from breast implants; for example, smoking cigarettes."[333]

Back in Midland, Michigan, Keith McKennon was busy preparing for a tidal wave of litigation. Even before the shock of a moratorium, Dow Corning had already suffered accelerating losses to the three pioneers of breast implant litigation: Robert Mithoff ($170,000), Nancy Hersh ($1.7 million), and Dan Bolton ($7.3 million). At the time of the Hopkins verdict, 137 cases were pending against the company. One month later, that number rose to 3,558. Dan Bolton alone received more than one thousand calls from worried women with implants; two hundred of them filed suits. Sidney Wolfe's Public Citizen Health Research Group was selling "How to Sue a Manufacturer" kits to registered trial lawyers for $750. One enterprising attorney offered free breast examinations to potential clients . . . seriously! But the company's greatest fear was mass tort litigation.[334]

Whenever a series of related injuries indicates that a multitude of victims might exist, the judicial system becomes vulnerable to a deluge of suits. English common law provided for the material interests of multiple damaged parties by registering them as a single class, thereby resolving their complaints with a single decree. In America, Rule 23 of the 1938 revision to the Federal Rules of Civil Procedure allowed for consolidation of closely related cases, registered by the judge as a class, along with appointment of a lead counsel empowered to choose one plaintiff who represents the entire class of litigants. The outcome of that single trial is applied to every other member of the class. Rule 23 was more often used to counteract injustices such as price rigging and civil rights violations. But in 1977, Cincinnati attorney Stanley Chesley pioneered use of the class action while litigating a Kentucky supper club fire that killed 166 people. After convincing the judge to declare all victims a single class, he conceived a novel legal theory: every manufacturer of potentially faulty aluminum wiring in the nation shared liability for damages regardless of whose product was used in the supper club. Suddenly, there were eleven hundred defendants facing one massive legal action with every defendant obligated to prove its innocence. If the lead plaintiff was ruled victorious, then all defendants shared the burden of an award driven by the emotions of the tragedy. Under these circumstances, it made better sense for the insurers to avoid a jury verdict and reach a pretrial financial agreement. Out of the forty-nine million dollar settlement pool generated, Chesley's firm took six million, a tidy sum by anyone's standard at the time. Stanley Chesley, in rewriting the strategy for successful injury litigation, established his reputation for all time.[335]

In 1983, Chesley began sparring with the Dow Chemical Company, the world's largest manufacturer of a dioxin-containing herbicide commonly referred to as Agent Orange. Dow's point man for the controversy was Keith McKennon. Chesley stunned the legal community when he achieved class certification for thousands of Vietnam War veterans, some with authenticated exposure and many more with presumed but unproven contact from its military use as a jungle defoliant. As the lone defendant, Dow Chemical faced as many as two hundred and fifty thousand claimants. Despite a lack of evidence linking Agent Orange to reported symptoms, the company agreed to pay one hundred and eighty million dollars for all existing suits in return for permanent protection from further dioxin litigation. McKennon was entirely comfortable with the company's one-time outlay; it was reasonable only when compared with the potential value of individual suits. Lawyers representing the litigants, on the other hand, were irate. The agreement limited awards to twelve thousand dollars per claimant regardless of disability. Attorneys were forced to extract their fees from that award while Chesley's firm collected five hundred and twenty five thousand dollars just to mediate the settlement. Despite the rancor, a precedent had been established for the trial bar: Agent Orange was the first class-action settlement for an alleged but unproven medical disability. It wouldn't be the last.[336]

Chesley's reputation for easy deal making came back to haunt him when he bullied his way into the breast implant litigation bonanza soon after the moratorium. Although he was a newcomer to the controversy, he was convinced he had the best answer, both for the plaintiffs and for corporate defendants that now included 3M, Baxter, and Bristol-Myers Squibb, each of whom acquired a small implant manufacturer during the decade prior to the controversy. Chesley was primarily Interested in the deepest pockets, not the small players like Inamed and Mentor. On January 24, 1992, he filed application for class certification in Cincinnati's Federal District Court where he could make his case before Judge Carl Rubin, who had approved the Agent Orange settlement. "These cases need some control, some direction to prevent chaos; you can't have thousands upon thousands of cases," he pleaded. The asbestos litigation, never consolidated, had been chaotic for the court system. The argument against consolidation was that each case deserved individual consideration; there was no common theme that joined Corley with Stern or Stern with Hopkins. Not persuaded, Rubin agreed to register the class for purposes of discovery only, ensuring that testimony from any witness would be immediately available to all other attorneys involved in breast implant litigation.

Trial attorneys throughout the nation howled in protest. Believing Chesley had previously sold out to Dow Chemical, Atlanta trial attorney Ralph Knowles wasn't shy about announcing where he stood: "I don't even know Chesley, but I have never seen such venom from so many plaintiff attorneys towards a fellow litigator." Knowles believed the spoils from breast implants amounted to billions of dollars not millions, and if they played their cards right, they could bring Dow Chemical in as a defendant even if it had never produced a single breast implant. "There was blood in the water and the sharks were circling," 3M defense counsel Joe Price later remarked.[337]

Dow Corning's McKennon had expected the class registration even before Rubin's decision and retained the services of Kenneth Feinberg, who had previously negotiated the Agent Orange agreement. Years later he would arbitrate distribution of funds to families of the World Trade Center victims and negotiate the BP Deepwater Horizon disaster settlement. Remembering him as being the best in the business, McKennon wanted Feinberg on his side of the table rather than on Chesley's team. But he had not anticipated Chesley losing the class to another federal district court. A breast implant task force was appointed by the Association of Trial Lawyers of America (ATLA) to more effectively resist Chesley, believing him to be on the side of big business. The matter was resolved by moving the class to Alabama's Federal District Judge Sam C. Pointer. Not willing to be displaced entirely from the enterprise, Chesley bought his way in by offering one million dollars of his firm's resources for a computer network to store every claim, every word of documentary evidence, every settlement offer and agreement, and all trial proceedings for every case within the court's jurisdiction. Judge Pointer was so impressed he appointed Chesley as cocounsel with Knowles.

No one was more critical of the notion of consolidating every breast implant victim into a single class than Houston's venerable John O'Quinn, known in Harris County, Texas, as the "Master of Disaster." His trial venue maintained standards of evidence far more favorable to plaintiffs plus higher payoffs to attorneys than any other state. Defense lawyers spoke of a "Texas premium" whenever jury awards were determined. Texas judges regularly stand for reelection and are accustomed to generous support from local attorneys. There was no more enthusiastic contributor to the political campaigns of Harris County judges than John O'Quinn, who believed he was, "blessed by God to help the little guy." Although his biggest awards totaling $1 billion were against Monsanto, Tenneco, and Amoco, he was especially proud of winning the largest verdict on behalf of an animal: $8.5 million for the wrongful death of a prized bull. O'Quinn and his partners Richard Laminack and Thomas Pirtle filed seventy-eight lawsuits on behalf of women with implants within a week of Dr. Kessler's announced moratorium. There would be hundreds more filed by Robert Mithoff, Michael Gallagher, and others during the months that followed. The Harris County Clerk later reported a backlog of two thousand breast implant cases.

The last thing that O'Quinn, Mithoff, or Gallagher wanted was a single class of implant suits under someone else's control. What O'Quinn did want was jurisdiction over all cases filed in the Texas state courts, where just a few enormous awards would justify the highest possible settlement price for their remaining clients. The most effective weapon for achieving this objective was a state law establishing that any suit filed against a citizen of Texas must be tried in the state court system and not in a federal court. Another Texas statute conveniently assigned partial liability for medical devices to the surgeon who implanted them. O'Quinn and his colleagues simply conamed the plastic surgeon in every breast case filed. And if that wasn't enough, they also listed Drs. Cronin and Gerow as inventors of a faulty device. By 1992, Dr. Cronin was retired and not in full command of his mental faculties. Family members later recalled how he responded politely to the doorbell, not fully comprehending the legal significance of subpoenas delivered to him by the hundreds.[338]

While Judge Pointer and the trial attorneys proceeded with their class action and the corporations deliberated over terms of a settlement, O'Quinn was looking for an ideal trial prospect, a plaintiff whose injury would assure a spectacular award. Preferring a defendant other than Dow Corning, he settled on Bristol-Myers Squibb, parent of Medical Engineering Corporation, the maker of implants used in 1976 to enlarge Pamela Johnson's breasts. O'Quinn reasoned that there was a clear advantage to battling a corporation defending itself on the basis of another company's research. His case was weak only because the client's symptoms were limited to modest fatigue following a rupture that required an implant replacement. He therefore needed to arouse the jury's sympathy for what might happen to her in the future. Texas colleagues admired O'Quinn for his Joe Six-Pack style; he could pronounce polydimethylsiloxane flawlessly, but he always referred to the polymer as "that stuff." Surgeons conamed in the suit could be relied on to support their patient's claim in return for having all charges against them dropped. This game was played time and again for every implant case tried in the state of Texas.[339]

Pamela Johnson's trial outcome would be determined by the testimony of Nir Kossovsky and that of opposing witness, Dr. Noel Rose. Without a degree in immunology, Kossovsky fancifully described the immune system as one set of toy soldiers battling another set. Rose, a distinguished professor of immunology at Johns Hopkins University, spoke with considerable authority when he said it was highly unlikely the plaintiff suffered any autoimmune disorder nor was she at risk of developing one in the future. Just as he had done in a 1990 letter to the FDA, he explained that adjuvant disease affected mice only when given a genuine adjuvant, that silicone by itself served no adjuvant role, and that there had never been a validated case of human adjuvant disease. During cross-examination, O'Quinn never challenged Rose's science. Instead, he quietly asked if the professor could understand the fears of women with silicone in their bodies? "I can understand but I'm not in that position myself," came his soft-spoken reply. When O'Quinn suggested that he was a lucky man, Rose unwittingly became the prosecution's star witness: "Indeed I am."[340]

The jury took less than four hours to issue a verdict on behalf of the plaintiff. Ms. Johnson sobbed as Judge Donald Wittig announced a recommended five million dollar compensatory award and twenty million in punitive damages. Once again, the trial captured the attention of all three network news anchors and dominated the next morning's headlines. Defense attorneys announced they would appeal, but in Texas they were unlikely to succeed. The Harris County Court Clerk registered five hundred more suits filed the following week. Bristol-Myers Squibb never tried another breast implant case, preferring to settle all claims for a rumored one million dollars per litigant. For O'Quinn, the victory was an important step in his grand plan: keep the awards as big as possible to sustain the highest possible settlement, perhaps rising to ten million dollars per client. But there was a downside to this kind of thinking; corporations, no matter how large they are, must define limits to what they can pay without declaring bankruptcy.[341]

As the year drew to a close, the harvest reaped by Commissioner Kessler's disposition of the breast implant issue included the following: 1). Several million anxious recipients of silicone devices, at least one million of them with breast implants; 2). Six thousand plaintiffs registered in state courts and four thousand in federal courts, each one convinced she was the unwitting victim of a defective product; 3). Virtually every plastic surgeon in the nation conamed in one or more implant suits; 4). Hundreds of plaintiff attorneys positioned to receive a 30–40 percent share of any award they might extract from a jury or a settlement conference; 5). Four major corporations and soon a fifth facing mass tort peril. The litigation juggernaut was now in command of events. When would science prevail?

13

DELIBERATING SCIENCE
IN THE COURTROOM

"In America, every political question . . . sooner or later . . .
becomes a judicial one."
—Alexis de Tocqueville[342]

"A trial is not a scientific inquiry into truth. A trial is merely
the resolution of a dispute.
—Edison Haines[343]

W hile French journalist Alexis de Tocqueville traveled
through America in 1830, he marveled that a newborn
republic's written laws and courts were not administered for the exclusive benefit of a limited aristocracy. Legal
advisory was accessible to ordinary citizens for settlement of disputes involving property and debts following divorce or death.
Tocqueville probably never imagined that a day would come when
questions of scientific validity would attract the scrutiny of the
nation's judiciary; the courtroom had never served as an effective
arena for debates of that kind, not in America, or Great Britain, or

France, or anywhere else. The issue that brought Galileo before the Holy Offices in Rome was heresy, not a precise definition of the cosmos.

Not until the nineteenth century was technology advanced sufficiently to influence everyday life experiences and thus become a judicial matter; yet the outcomes of these deliberations were often confounding. Without valid definitions of mental status, questions of sanity in the courtroom were stymied. Following the death of President James Garfield in 1881, the jury relied on the simple facts before them: Garfield was dead and Charles Guiteau was his admitted assassin. Deliberating for one hour, the jury declared the defendant guilty of first-degree murder and promptly hanged him. The 1925 trial of a schoolteacher, John T. Scopes, for teaching Darwinian evolutionary principles continues to epitomize judicial confusion whenever science conflicts with biblical teaching.[344]

In a modern age characterized by unrelenting technological advances, the resolution of legal disputes involving human safety requires a contemporary understanding of natural and physical laws. Members of the legal profession are not often prepared academically for this challenge. What they are deft with is the process of negotiation, but science is not based on collaboration or consensus. Its laws, once revealed, are firm unless challenged with new evidence; no jury should ever have to vote on whether a whale is a mammal or a fish. Furthermore, scientists and attorneys approach their respective duties from opposing directions. In the laboratory or the clinic, the investigator's conclusions evolve from a consideration of all available evidence. Lawyers on the other hand work from a desired outcome and then offer only the evidence that supports their client's best interest. The courtroom, therefore, is the last place a learned man would choose to resolve a scientific conflict. Yet with increasing frequency, questions of scientific validity are often seen on dockets throughout the nation.[345]

Accusations of wrongful injury have long been a fertile field for argumentation requiring expert testimony. Legal authority for resolving personal injury disputes was established in America during the mid-nineteenth century with the writing of tort laws. A tort is a civil violation as opposed to a criminal act. For the first time, private individuals could sue for damages inflicted by a "tortfeasor," meaning anyone who has committed a noncriminal injury. In its broadest scope, the law of torts encompasses libel, slander, and trespass of property, but for the most part, early tort actions arose from accidents and physical injuries. During the late 1800s, there were few circumstances that more grotesquely mauled a body than hot coals spewing from a speeding locomotive or the exploding boiler of a steamboat. Early applications of tort law therefore grew out of a powerful engine's deforming impact on the unprotected laborer. At first, victims of industrial accidents rarely prevailed against the mighty railroads defended by attorneys educated in the nation's finest law schools. Their claims failed to even reach the court docket. Eventually, tort actions became the province of a different class of attorneys, the brightest sons of immigrant families who after laboring all day, studied law at night, and with dogged persistence graduated with law degrees. For these scrappy lawyers and their hopeful clients, success in the form of a monetary award required a trial and a jury verdict favorable to the injured party. Advocates of tort victims thus became known as trial lawyers, and when they established a trade association, they called it the Association of Trial Lawyers of America (ATLA).[346]

Because laborers could not afford to pay up front for legal services, their attorneys accepted the risk and collected a percentage of any award resulting from their efforts. A system of fees paid on contingency was born of necessity with the concurrence of judicial authorities. Because the best interests of the trial lawyers were often dependent on their political ties, ATLA members established the habit of contributing mightily to local and national campaigns. Even today, the association contributes a greater percentage of its operating budget to support of candidates than most other trade organizations.[347]

Plaintiffs and trial attorneys have never had an easy time fighting large corporations. According to the common law principle of strict liability, proof of negligence was required before an employer was found culpable for payment of damages. Strict liability was eventually replaced by moral liability, which obligates a manufacturer to provide safe working conditions and a product that is not defective. Furthermore, whenever risks are known in advance—for example, a drug side effect or a device complication—the manufacturer is obligated to warn of risks.[348]

Tort law in the twentieth century has been applied broadly to all potential hazards resulting from the use of any manufactured product. For example, tort actions were filed soon after the alleged horrors of elixir sulfanilamide, Thalidomide, and the Dalkon Shield were revealed. So there should have been no surprise when lawyers nationwide seized the opportunity to litigate for damages resulting from breast implants, especially after an agency of government questioned their safety.

Despite unprecedented awards in San Francisco and Houston, success for plaintiffs, as well as for defendants, was dependent on the evidence available at trial and how it was presented. Harris County jurors were not capable of distinguishing the speculative theories of a UCLA pathologist from the carefully articulated opinion of a Johns Hopkins immunologist. But trials in the future offered a different prospect, especially if the attorneys or the experts or the evidence underwent constructive transformation. Faced with hundreds of new filings every day, Keith McKinnon replaced Frank Woodside with David M. Bernick as Dow Corning's national trial counsel. Woodside's fate was limited to taking depositions from opponent witnesses.[349]

Bernick, a highly successful litigator for the Chicago defense firm Kirkland & Ellis, had previously demonstrated his aptitude for tackling complex scientific issues in the courtroom. "My basic premise is that jurors can understand science if you take the time to explain it to them." He studied philosophy at the University of Chicago but didn't recognize his capacity for mastering the complexities of technology until he chose law for a career. Working on behalf of Dow Chemical, he successfully defended a pesticide falsely linked with neurological disease. Later, he established the innocence of "Sarabond," a chemical additive used in construction mortar, saving Dow more than one hundred million dollars in claims. One Dow executive later said, "To call Dave Bernick brilliant is an understatement."[350]

Watching a television report of the Mariann Hopkins award, Bernick imagined himself reversing Dow Corning's ill fortune as he had once done for Dow Chemical. After convincing the company that their opponent's weakness was a faulty scientific theory, he immersed himself in silicone polymer chemistry, biomaterials science, and autoimmune disease. Next he prepared himself to counter the dubious testimony of each and every plaintiff expert. He recruited the best experts he could find from academia, national agencies, and corporate laboratories. Bernick believed the science available to him was better than any prior defense counsels had made use of. The 1950 toxicology experiments completed by V. K. Rowe had established the remarkable biologic compatibility of silicone polymers, but this important laboratory precedent had not been shown to any jury. The studies of Munson and White demonstrating silicone's negligible immune reactivity had been passed over by defense attorneys. The experiments conducted by Rudolph showing little consequence from microscopic gel bleed had never been explained in any courtroom.[351]

Bernick established an effective collaboration with epidemiologist Ralph Cook, who had compiled the pertinent evidence derived from population studies. Both were reassured by new findings. Canadians are disciplined record keepers just like their British forebears; the Province of Alberta was capable of tracking the health status of all its citizens, among them eleven thousand recipients of breast implants. Drawing from the health department's database and tumor registry, University of Calgary plastic surgeon Dale Birdsell and Alberta Cancer Board epidemiologist Hans Berkel joined to complete a nonconcurrent cohort linkage study showing that women with breast implants were no more likely to develop breast cancer than those without. Theirs proved to be the long-awaited confirmation of the Los Angeles–USC findings.

Even more important to David Bernick than the publication of corroborative evidence favorable to the company's position was finding additional databases available for examining issues other than cancer risk. The Nurses Health database at Harvard's School of Public Health contained health information from one hundred and twenty thousand nurses, allowing for study of specific patterns and causes of disease. The Mayo Clinic had long rendered care to patients from all over the world but also to nearly every resident of surrounding Olmsted County. The medical records of 4.3 million citizens who had lived in the county since 1907 represented another database for the conduct of cohort studies.[352]

David Bernick's first opportunity to defend Dow Corning came in May 1993. Denver plaintiff Tammy Turner-McCartney, a part-time topless dancer, acknowledged that her implants had helped her professionally but also believed they made her sick. Her case was not a compelling one because extensive diagnostic surveys failed to reveal any specific illness. Nonetheless, her attorney accepted the risk of a costly trial. Bernick prepared himself to defend not only Dow Corning's record of advancing technology but also its standards of corporate conduct. He coached his company witnesses with great care, each of them schooled in the abundant research Dow Corning had previously conducted or sponsored. To his jury, he explained that leakage of silicone from implants was a known and accepted property of all permeable membranes and not a product defect. Dow Corning's device, he added, retained its gel as well as any other manufacturer's product. Furthermore, the quantity of seepage was visible to an electron microscope and nothing like the spreading ink blot portrayed on television screens. During cross-examination of the plaintiff, Bernick asked about a motor vehicle accident prior to her implants. She had blamed her injury for the same complaints she was now attributing to her breast surgery.[353]

The linchpin of Dow Corning's defense, however, was Bernick's handling of the plaintiff's experts. Pierre Blais, a chemist by training, was effectively discredited when forced to admit he had never conducted silicone research in any laboratory or clinic.

Furthermore, he was not a physician and agreed he was not qualified to offer medical opinions. Another expert, Andrew Campbell,
operated a chronic fatigue clinic in Houston but admitted under
cross-examination that he had fraudulently added to his resumé
several professional affiliations in fields like immunology and toxicology. He wasn't qualified for any of them. Neither was he aware
of the plaintiff's prior auto accident. Campbell's career as a witness for trial lawyers was finished.

The defense verdict that followed was Dow Corning's first
breast implant trial victory. Local reporters immediately branded
the jury's decision a biased condemnation of the plaintiff's public
nudity. Just as quickly, jury foreman Charles Van Devander issued
a sharply worded rebuttal that appeared in the *Rocky Mountain
News*. The plaintiff's work history was never an issue in determining the outcome, he declared. "What was wrong with her case was
that her attorneys could not prove that implants caused any illness.
The easiest way to explain the verdict was that the plaintiff had
very little evidence, and all the evidence presented was effectively
rebutted by the defense."[354]

The Denver verdict was followed a few weeks later by a similar victory in Colorado Springs. Was the tide suddenly turning in
favor of Dow Corning and other manufacturers as well? Buttressed
by two epidemiologic studies, the cancer issue no longer served as
the litigation threat it had once been. As for rheumatic disease,
the message was clear that juries were now demanding evidence
of genuine illness, not just fatigue and aches and pains. The
Colorado trial outcomes didn't escape the notice of every attorney
in the nation caught up in the breast litigation whirlwind, including cocounsels Knowles and Chesley and the Texas group led by
John O'Quinn. Product liability defense attorneys began preparing their cases more carefully. On their own, Knowles and Chesley
met secretly with Feinberg about a settlement. Other trial lawyers
were incensed when the news leaked. Knowles was forced to apol-
ogize for his treachery.

Houston attorney Mike Gallagher, with more than a thousand breast implant cases filed, became the new watchdog for

what was now called the Plaintiff's Steering Committee. Unlike O'Quinn, Gallagher believed that a strategy based on steadily increasing awards would lead inevitably to the insolvency of one or more corporations. Bankrupting the deep pockets wasn't in the best interest of anyone. And so it came to pass that under a Texas lawyer's direct influence, the pace of settlement negotiations accelerated.[355]

Defense attorneys were stunned by Gallagher's audacity when they learned what he was demanding: each claimant must have an opportunity to opt out of the settlement if their payoff (not yet calculable) proved insufficient. Neither did he believe plaintiffs should have to prove disease causation. Even if a victim's symptoms failed to match those of any recognizable disease, Gallagher insisted on the woman's right to make a claim. And so the Steering Committee introduced the concept of atypical disease, maladies not yet recognized by medical science. Disorders of the nervous system, none of them appearing in any textbook, eventually appeared on the claim eligibility list.[356]

In September 1993, the four major implant manufacturers—Dow Corning, Bristol-Myers Squibb, Baxter Healthcare, and 3M—jointly announced they had collectively set aside $4.75 billion to settle claims filed over the next thirty years. Dow Corning's share was approximately two billion. Trial lawyers would receive for their services 25 percent of the payoff, something in excess of one billion dollars, and all of it up front rather than over a span of decades. Estimated payments for individual plaintiffs ranged from two hundred thousand dollars to two million depending on the disability. Two implant manufacturers, Inamed and Mentor, declined, threatening bankruptcy instead. Taking them at their word, the committee accepted smaller settlements.[357]

The agreement was soon labeled the "global settlement" because its jurisdiction included claims as far away as Australia, where Dow Corning dominated the implant market. Skeptics believed the agreement was structured to fail, its major flaw being the indeterminate claimant pool. Without knowing how many would seek their pot of gold, it was impossible to estimate the size of individual awards. Eighteen thousand had already filed; Feinberg's negotiating team imagined there might be as many as sixty thousand. If there were more, the payoffs diminished and claimants held the right to opt out and sue anyway.[358]

Nancy Hersh, whose litigation had produced one of the earliest jury verdicts against the breast implant, believed the class action would attract the wrong kind of people, meaning women who had not been harmed by implants. Still convinced that her client was sick and had deserved her award, Hersh would have nothing to do with the global settlement. "I don't like people who live off us; they are making an industry out of women's injuries."[359]

Meanwhile, John O'Quinn and his partners were busy preparing their cases and winning awards as high as nineteen million dollars. Because he was filing in the Texas court system, O'Quinn was not restricted by the global settlement or by any judicial decisions coming from Alabama. His simple answer to fears that the settlement might eventually unravel was to bring another deep pocket into the sphere of legal vulnerability. His target was Dow Chemical with annual revenues of $20 billion, ten times larger than Dow Corning. Judge Pointer had previously ruled that Dow Chemical was not a producer of breast implants and therefore free of culpability. But O'Quinn's research had revealed that the company had conducted toxicology studies on behalf of Dow Corning during the 1940s; furthermore, the two companies had jointly produced a pesticide containing silicone. It was a tenuous linkage but it was enough evidence for a Texas judge to qualify Dow Chemical as a defendant in breast implant litigation.

O'Quinn promptly filed against both Midland companies on behalf of two carefully selected plaintiffs, Gladys Laas, a matronly fifty-seven-year-old who suffered chronic breast pain, and Jenny Ladner, a thirty-five-year-old physician afflicted with systemic lupus erythematosus. Dow Chemical's calculated response was to sue Dow Corning, a tactical maneuver to secure its cooperation and all of its research data. But what Dow executives really wanted was the services of David Bernick, who promptly agreed. Although teams of attorneys would work on behalf of their respective clients, what this case featured for the first time was Bernick and O'Quinn engaged in courtroom combat.[360]

While he was preparing for trial, Bernick learned of newly published evidence that strengthened his client's position. From the M. D. Andersen Cancer Center in Houston came a survey of six hundred mastectomy patients, half of them reconstructed with silicone implants and the other half repaired with flaps of their own tissue. The incidence of autoimmune disease was both negligible and identical in each group. While it didn't qualify as an epidemiologic study, its source was a celebrated Texas institution known to any potential juror. And there was another timely gift for the defense, the awaited cohort study from the Mayo Clinic. Epidemiologist Sherine Gabriel reported in the *New England Journal of Medicine,* that she had found "no association between breast implants and connective tissue diseases or other similar disorders" among 794 Olmsted County women living in apparent harmony with their breast implants for as long as thirty years. In an accompanying editorial, Gabriel's work was declared scientifically meticulous and sorely needed, but readers were also cautioned that negative studies are never the final word. Trial lawyers naturally focused on the caveats instead of the findings.[361]

But there was even more for Bernick to exploit and O'Quinn to worry about. Preliminary findings derived from the Harvard Nurses's Study had surfaced as a prepublication abstract showing no association between breast implants and any recognized rheumatic illness. O'Quinn did all he could to keep this information out of the impending trial. The Mayo study was not definitive, he argued; even the journal's editor said so. And the Harvard study hadn't even been published yet. Bernick insisted the evidence was both authentic and deserved a hearing. In a compromise ruling, the judge agreed to admit the Mayo Clinic findings because they had appeared in a medical journal, but the Harvard study wasn't published so "its findings will not be heard in this courtroom . . . end of argument!"[362]

In sharp contrast to O'Quinn's larger-than-life presence, Bernick was barely visible from behind his podium but he left no doubt in any juror's mind that he believed his opponent held no credible evidence proving his client's product had caused any disease process. Bernick carefully avoided any challenge of the illnesses reported by the two plaintiffs. Instead, he based his case on the faulty testimony of O'Quinn's experts. Campbell and Blais were of course out of the picture. Kossovsky, however, was back, this time with a laboratory test, Detecsil, for what he claimed were immune reactions to silicone. Under cross-examination, the UCLA pathologist agreed that of two hundred and fifty women claiming illness, only two reacted to his test. And he was forced to admit that testing of samples sent to him from the Scripps Clinic had failed to distinguish women with and without silicone exposure.[363]

Bernick kept using O'Quinn's own witnesses against him. Dr. Thomas Biggs, longstanding partner in the Cronin Plastic Surgery Group, testified that Dow Corning had not been straight-forward in its communications with surgeons about the fragility of mammary devices. O'Quinn also highlighted the surgeon's willingness to provide testimony without charge. Under cross, Bernick elicited from Biggs that he never told patients that implants caused immune disease. Biggs added that he knew of no reports proving that any immune disease was caused by medical grade silicone. When Bernick revisited the matter of testifying without a fee, the doctor acknowledged he had been conamed in the suit and that the charges were since dropped. A skilled defense attorney had just revealed a witness "testifying to save his own skin."[364]

John O'Quinn had wanted his case to be about morality and ethics, but his opponent had forced a consideration of polymer chemistry and medical science. Summarizing his case on behalf of Dow Corning, Bernick asked, "Where in all the closing arguments from Mr. O'Quinn today did you hear reference to a single study?" When the foreman was asked for the outcome, he issued one of the most confounding verdicts in breast implant litigation history. For one plaintiff he declared the companies innocent of all wrongdoing. For the second, the jury concluded that Dow Corning had not acted negligently, had not produced a defective device, and had not misinformed its clients about the device. Yet they found both companies guilty of "deceptive trade practices," and for this an award of $5.2 million was to be shared by all defendants including Dow Chemical. No punitive damages were assigned. Not even John O'Quinn could make sense of the verdict. The judge later vacated the ruling against Dow Chemical because it was incompatible with the remainder of the verdict, making the victory more important for Dow Chemical than for its Midland subsidiary. The chemical giant was not yet obliged to join the ranks of global settlement contributors.

As for Dow Corning, its qualified victory in Texas was meaningless in practical terms because time was running out. The claimant pool had risen to four hundred and eighty thousand, unimagined to negotiators at the time of the settlement. Nearly all were free of disease or even symptoms, but Dow Corning was still worried about what might lie ahead. Faced with a landslide of financial obligations, Judge Pointer declared the global settlement underfunded by at least three billion dollars. If this wasn't enough of a burden for the corporations to bear, they faced another six thousand cases filed in Harris County where O'Quinn was securing awards or settlements averaging thirteen million dollars. A CPA wasn't needed to estimate the calamity that Dow Corning faced.

On May 15, 1995 in Bay City, Michigan, Dow Corning President Gary Anderson filed for Chapter 11 bankruptcy protection, thus placing all of Dow Corning's litigation on hold and canceling its two billion dollar obligation to Judge Pointer. In his statement, Anderson cited the irony of "all this happening now just as the science is saying there is no connection between the implants and the immune-system diseases that are alleged here." Not since A. H. Robins succumbed to more than two hundred thousand Dalkon Shield claims had there been as large a bankruptcy involving a medical product. Most plastic surgeons were stunned, failing to understand how a major corporation could speak of a "wise business decision." Few people realized that Dow Corning had already paid out one hundred and eighty million dollars in legal defense costs and even worse, its corporate insurers were balking at the prospect of having to make restitution for these costs.[365]

Sybil Goldrich, who had promised her dying mother she would "move on," meaning take up some cause other than breast implants, proudly announced: "I look forward to serving as a trustee for the Dow Corning bankruptcy . . . that is my dream. That company now belongs to the women it injured." How did the nation's trial lawyers respond to the bankruptcy? They refiled their Dow Corning suits, every one of them, but this time they named Dow Chemical as codefendant. The chemical giant's Texas victory proved to be a temporary escape; it would endure many more days in court.

Most corporations are protected by a phalanx of insurers, each assuming risk for one segment of their liability. When 3M surveyed the position of each of its insurers, it discovered that most were refusing to compensate the company for implant losses. Insurance underwriters, like end users, expect to be informed in advance of any risk potential. Their basis for withholding payment was a belief that manufacturers failed to inform them of known dangers. A prolonged standoff ensued that led to countless hearings and trials over a span of many years. The ruling came from a single judge, not a jury, and insurers were forced to meet their obligations; manufacturers had not hidden their risks. Meanwhile, years of delay protected insurers' assets, placing additional financial strain on manufacturers.[366]

In the midst of the litigation frenzy, a group of Texas plastic surgeons led by Dr. Simon Fredericks took the position that they had suffered financially at the hands of sixteen derelict implant manufacturers just as their many patients had suffered medically. In their filing of *Levine et al. v. Bristol-Myers Squibb (BMS) et al.*, they sought compensation for damages resulting from diminished practice revenue, from time spent dealing with angry patients, and from the stress of multiple legal actions brought against them. In what became known as "the doctors' suit," Dr. Fredericks avoided the salvos of defense attorneys; that fate would befall San Antonio plastic surgeon Richard Levine, who unwittingly permitted his name to appear first among the plaintiffs. Attorneys from Shook, Hardy & Bacon, a Kansas City firm famous for its aggressive defense of the tobacco industry and counsel for lead defendant Bristol-Myers Squibb, demanded from Dr. Levine not only his financial records but also his personal health records documenting emotional stress, as well as confidential records of several hundred patients. Except for major legal costs on both sides, *Levine v. BMS* never went anywhere. None of the surgeons involved had foreseen that the discovery process could penetrate their professional and personal lives. Except for adding to the balance sheets of all attorneys involved, nothing positive came from *Levine vs. BMS*.[367]

In another large state, members of the California Society of Plastic Surgeons collaborated with The Doctor's Company, a professional liability underwriter, to form a defense strategy based entirely on scientific evidence demonstrating safety for every kind of silicone medical device. A team of defense attorneys was prepped using mock trials with multiple panels of jurors, all of them interviewed and their impressions tabulated. No California plastic surgeon suffered indemnity for diseases alleged to follow use of breast implants. Trial attorneys preferred as targets corporations with much deeper pockets.

Testifying before a House of Representatives subcommittee just three months after public notice of Dow Corning's bankruptcy, Commissioner Kessler suddenly announced, "We now have, for the first time, a reasonable assurance that silicone-gel implants do not cause a large increase in traditional connective-tissue disease in women." He failed to cite the evidence that led the agency to alter its position. Without a press release following his testimony, his statement never appeared in any FDA publication, so the press paid no attention. Trial attorneys, meanwhile, continued to pin their hopes on his reference to "traditional connective tissue disease." Why? Because the Plaintiff's Steering Committee was still hoping for recognition of the "atypical connective tissue diseases."[368]

Kessler's own staff supported that effort by cosponsoring with NIH a consensus workshop, "Atypical Rheumatic Diseases and Silicone Breast Implants," thus implying that a new category of illness merely required a committee to establish a definition. Workshop organizers Lori Brown and Louise Brinton were defiantly resistant to the protestations of experts representing the American College of Rheumatology, who gave no meaning to any disease that lacked measurable and reproducible diagnostic criteria. In other words, an elusive atypical connective disease served only as fodder for existing litigation and did not even qualify for study using epidemiologic methods.[369]

The following lessons should have been clear at this point. First, the mere absence of a proven cause for damages resulting from exposure to any manufactured product cannot ward off mass tort litigation. Second, regulatory agencies such as the FDA cannot be expected to back down or admit error, regardless of the power of new evidence. And third, neither trial lawyers nor corporate attorneys will make use of all the evidence that bears on a scientific question. What was still required for clarity and justice was the courage of a judge willing to distinguish between good evidence and bad. For the silicone controversy, that person was Robert E. Jones of the U. S. District Court in Portland, Oregon, who famously applied a recent Supreme Court decision, then appointed his own panel of scientific experts, and proceeded to transform forever the rules applicable to breast implant litigation.

All legal proceedings are governed by established rules of evidence. For cases involving scientific issues, *Frye vs. United States* became the prevailing standard in 1923 when the District of Columbia Circuit Court of Appeals decided a lie detector test was admissible in a criminal trial. Justices also ruled that the scientific community was best qualified to define its own standard. The *Frye* test, as it came to be known, required that scientific evidence be "generally accepted" by those who practice within a "particular field." Critics later claimed the test was ambiguous and restrictive. A "particular field" is often hard to define because the boundaries of scientific disciplines are changing all the time. Neither is "generally accepted" easily defined. The need for a scientific consensus might exclude groundbreaking discoveries not yet recognized. Worst of all, *Frye* encouraged judges to abdicate their responsibility for evaluating the reliability of experts testifying in their courtrooms. Nonetheless, *Frye* remained the accepted standard for the next seventy years.[370]

Attorneys for both a plaintiff and a defendant understand the influence that any expert witness can exert on the opinions of jurors, whether or not the testimony is legitimate. Juries are easily confused whenever distinctions between authentic and false expertise are cloudy. The typical juror is particularly vulnerable to hindsight bias, meaning a tendency to judge prior incidents according to a known outcome. People who are unaware of an outcome can more easily avoid such bias. But jurors are nearly always informed of an outcome during opening arguments, and they will use that foreknowledge as a shortcut to decision making. For example, in cases of toxic exposure, the easiest decision is to link the reported effect with the alleged cause, especially when a phony expert is brought forward to promote the notion. All valid scientific evidence to the contrary is more than likely rejected. Only a judge is in a position to control hindsight bias by ensuring the highest standard of evidence offered at trial.[371]

In 1975, the *Frye* test was displaced by new rules of evidence written for the purpose of redefining the eligibility of expert witnesses. Rules 104 and 706 (1975) broadened the admissibility of expert testimony, but the outcome was unfortunate. Experts with dubious expertise descended on courtrooms with countless unproven theories. The *Frye* test therefore persisted in several states until 1984 when litigation filed in San Diego called attention to a conflict between the two existing standards. The circumstances of the case were remarkably similar to where breast implant litigation stood at about the same time. Following a pregnancy marked by persistent nausea, Jason Daubert was born with congenital deformities involving his right extremity. His mother had taken the antihistamine Bendectin throughout her pregnancy to control vomiting. After her son's birth, hindsight bias led a jury to blame Bendectin for the deformities. In a suit filed against manufacturer Merrell Dow Pharmaceuticals, attorneys for the plaintiff sought more liberal rules while defense attorneys insisted on the longstanding *Frye* test. Siding with the defense, the judge disallowed anecdotes from plaintiff experts and admitted the available epidemiologic studies. A defense verdict followed that was later upheld by the Ninth District Federal Court of Appeals. Meanwhile, the unresolved question of competing evidentiary standards was taken to the U. S. Supreme Court for resolution.[372]

In *Daubert v. Merrell Dow Pharmaceuticals Inc. (1993)*, the Supreme Court sidestepped the question of Bendectin causing birth defects and focused on standards for admissibility of scientific evidence at trial. Because of the importance of the case, amicus briefs were filed by scientific journals such as the *New England Journal of Medicine* in support of the more restrictive *Frye standard*. Writing for the majority, Justice Harry Blackmun went beyond *Frye* by giving judges "a gatekeeper function ensuring that all scientific evidence admitted in testimony was both relevant and reliable." Four possible considerations for determining reliability were listed: 1) Has the expert's theory been tested; is it even capable of being tested? 2) What are the testing parameters? 3) Has the expert's methodology been subjected to peer-review and publication? 4) Has the expert's theory been accepted by the scientific community?[373]

Spokesmen for the American Bar Association and the American Association for the Advancement of Science were jubilant. In their eyes, the Supreme Court had embraced the convictions of Karl Popper, who believed that the key to proving a scientific theory was its "falsifiability." A theory is worthy of consideration only if it can be tested and either corroborated or rejected, which is exactly what Justice Blackmun expected of judges facing issues dependent upon scientific evidence. But where could judges be found who were equipped to serve the gatekeeper function? If they existed they were rare, according to critics of the decision. It soon fell to the justices of the Ninth Circuit to demonstrate their own willingness to face the challenge that *Daubert* presented to the judiciary.[374]

Only by coincidence did the Bendectin case return to San Francisco for reconsideration at a time when the appeal of *Hopkins v. Dow Corning* was due for Ninth Circuit review. *Hopkins* was the first opportunity for an appellate court to apply the *Daubert* instruction; regrettably the outcome was far short of visionary. Appellate justices found the testimony of all experts in *Hopkins* to be admissible and affirmed the verdict. But a few months later the same court ruled in favor of Bendectin and its manufacturer. It was sufficient precedent to grant promise for defusing the influence that dubious experts impose on trial outcomes.[375]

What became known simply as *Daubert* attracted the interest of Judge Robert Jones when he was faced with *Hall v. Baxter Healthcare,* the first of several breast implant cases crowding his court docket. Despite longstanding promises from Judge Pointer to appoint experts, Jones tired of waiting and became the first judge to apply *Daubert* to breast implant litigation. For his own panel of experts, he appointed a polymer chemist, an immunologist, a rheumatologist, and an epidemiologist, then asked them to advise the court on each designated expert's proposed testimony.[376]

More than a year had passed since David Bernick and John O'Quinn squared off in a Houston courtroom, and during that interval, even more evidence had become available for the Jones panel to review. Now in the public domain were the results of additional follow-up using Harvard's databases. Following a review of records from 87,501 women, there was still no identifiable association between breast implants and connective tissue disease. It was the largest cohort study to date; yet it failed to generate much press notice. The results were presented in terms of relative risk, a mathematical expression not easily grasped by reporters, newspaper readers, television viewers, or jurors.[377]

At about the same time, another group of enterprising investigators assembled every known scientific publication dealing with the breast implant issue—twenty-six hundred in all! Thirteen of these reports were considered eligible for "meta-analysis," a sophisticated test of statistical significance already popular with epidemiologists. Meta-analysis involves the consolidation of several studies into one in order to test theories using a larger population for greater statistical power. Once again, no causal links between breast implants and any rheumatic disease were identified. Regrettably, Ralph Cook, who led the team performing this meta-analysis, was employed by Dow Corning and nobody at the time was willing to believe anything Dow Corning had to say.[378]

The Harvard study and Cook's meta-analysis were, however, available to Judge Jones' panel, along with a recent report from the British Medical Device Directorate deciding once again that no evidence existed to support a link between connective tissue diseases and breast implants. After four days of hearings, the Jones panel concluded that "any theory supporting a claim alleging linkage between breast implants and any autoimmune disease was at best an untested hypothesis." Suddenly, the rules for conducting breast implant litigation changed. *Daubert* hearings to evaluate the qualifications of listed expert witnesses became a familiar preliminary to any trial. Ruled inadmissible in many jurisdictions was all testimony from Marc Lappe, Pierre Blais, and Nir Kossovsky and, in time, many more of the trial attorneys' stable of experts.[379]

The last thing that Knowles or Chesley wanted was a thorough examination of the scientific evidence. Judge Pointer, on the other hand, faced his own duty under the *Daubert* ruling and could procrastinate no longer. Managing to find four experts without prior involvement with medical device manufacturers or breast implant litigations, he demanded the steering committee's reluctant approval and appointed what came to be known as the National Science Panel. But instead of performing inside of a few weeks as Jones' panel had done, Pointer's experts took another two years to issue its report. Anticipating that the findings would not favor their cause, Knowles accused the panel of being "tainted by industry money." A lone member had years before received a $750 honorarium from Bristol-Myers Squibb for participating in a company-sponsored symposium. Because the accused was from Ottawa, Canada, and in no way a party to any part of an American controversy, Judge Pointer overruled the complaint and let the report stand. Its conclusion was both clear and decisive: "Silicone gel breast implants do not precipitate novel immune responses, nor induce systemic inflammation, nor alter the severity of any autoimmune disease."[380]

The National Science Panel experience provided some practical lessons for the federal judiciary. First, all such expert panels can be very expensive. Experts must be compensated for taking lengthy blocks of time away from their primary responsibilities. Second, recruiting truly "independent" authorities without prior industry ties is a daunting task and won't become any easier in the future. Third, science panels are inherently inefficient and emotionally bruising. When members of Pointer's panel reflected on their experience, they spoke of rude cross-examinations during their confirmation, repeated insults, and ad hominem attacks coming from the steering committee throughout. Conversations among them were restricted. And they were all deposed at the end to determine how they had reached their conclusions. The federal judiciary has work to do if it expects to be served by the nation's most-qualified authorities.[381]

As the end of the 1990s approached, the defendant corporations were no longer as vulnerable to the awards that captured headlines earlier in the decade. Except for an occasional defendant unwilling to relinquish her day in court, trials were less frequent and settlements diminished as evidence mounted that silicone was not the cause of any disease.

In 1999, two government-sponsored bodies weighed in on the controversy. The British Medical Device Directorate, at the urging of Parliament where a few members were sympathetic to increasingly vocal activists, reviewed the evidence once more with no change in its prior conclusions. And at the urging of the U. S. House of Representatives, The Institute of Medicine (IOM) issued its own appraisal of breast implants.[382]

Under the chairmanship of University of North Carolina Professor of Medicine Stuart Bondurant, thirteen medical scientists devoted two years to the most exacting survey of its kind yet completed. In sharp contrast to the formal scientific proceedings held at the National Academy of Sciences, the IOM hearings were often unruly, just as FDA hearings had been in the past; members of the same activist groups attended in force and were characteristically vocal with their own version of the truth. The panel focused on the same old questions: Were any of the materials used in the devices toxic to humans? Was the immune system affected? Were claims of a connective tissue disease meritorious? Did women with breast implants who nursed place their offspring at risk?[383]

In its final report released on June 21, 1999, the IOM panel declared invalid all claims of carcinogenic, mutagenic, teratogenic, or immunologic influence. The available toxicological evidence for silicone polymer safety in experimental animals and in humans was substantial and convincing, even at challenge doses far greater than would be experienced by women with breast implants. Traces of platinum and nickel in silicone devices were determined to be inconsequential. Their conviction applied to recent allegations of mysterious soft tissue sarcomas resulting from breast implantation, aggressively pushed by the Plaintiff's Steering Committee. And the panel was not buying the notion of an "atypical silicone disease," long promoted by trial attorneys and the FDA.[384]

Breast implants did not receive a totally clean bill of health from the IOM. In addition to citing the long-recognized local complications including firm breasts, rupture, and deflation, the report emphasized that women should anticipate reoperation for correction of these undesired outcomes. Agreeing that manufacturers were continually improving their products, the panel challenged the industry to pursue better methods for identifying rupture in the absence of symptoms, and to conduct more studies to determine whether mammography delayed breast cancer diagnosis.[385]

The report's 415 pages of interpretation, recommendations, and bibliography left no pending issue unstudied. It would stand as the most authoritative confirmation of silicone as the safest available biomaterial for nonrigid (meaning nonmetallic) devices. Yet, news reporting of the Institute's findings was difficult to find. Unlike a record-breaking punitive damage award, it wasn't the

kind of story that news anchors sought for their evening broadcast or that an editor wanted to devote column space to. Print
journalists and the broadcast media had nearly abandoned breast
implants and turned to more compelling issues. More newswor-
thy at the time was the prospect of electromagnetic waves causing
brain cancer. As for the trial lawyers who knew the IOM report
was coming, they were moving on to more lucrative opportunities.

For those with continuing exposure to an implanted silicone device, most had already decided the risk was small and
were proceeding with their lives. The few women who remained
convinced they were victims of a toxic material were not about
to change their position or their habits; for them, all authorities
including the IOM were merely apologists for the breast implant
industry. Meanwhile, the IOM published a reassuring booklet for
consumers optimistically titled, "Information for Women About
the Safety of Silicone Breast Implants." But not the FDA; its website continued for years after to list connective tissue disease as a
risk of breast implants. It wasn't easy or common for an agency of
government to change its mind.[386]

14

SCIENCE, REGULATION, AND THE POLITICS OF RISK

"In framing a government to be administered by men over men,
first enable the government to control the governed;
then oblige it to control itself."
—James Madison, *The Federalist #51*[387]

B y the time the Institute of Medicine granted its 1999 pardon
to the embattled breast implant, a decade had passed since
Public Citizen's Sidney Wolfe issued his dire prophecy: an
epidemic of cancer afflicting thousands of unsuspecting women
harboring the devices. Allegations of more than two hundred silicone-induced symptoms or illnesses followed his unsubstantiated
warning. During the years that followed, no such plague ensued
nor was any illness linked to silicone exposure. In the meantime,
more than eleven billion dollars (fifteen billion in today's dollars)
was spent by medical device makers to preserve their commercial

viability and appease the fugitive demands of America's litigation industry. Three manufacturers of breast implants had either
declared bankruptcy or discontinued their medical product lines,
while four major corporations with device subsidiaries terminat-
ed their engagement with silicone medical products. Implantable
device innovation in America had nearly come to a standstill, and
for the first time silicone product development gained traction in
Europe and Asia.

All the while, several million people with appropriately
functioning silicone devices in place remained in doubt about
the safety of their devices. Women with breast implants, most of
them still enthusiastic about the outcomes of their surgery, were
nonetheless disturbed by persistent media reminders of the tragic consequences that might lie ahead. Thousands more awaited
compensation for injuries they alone attributed to silicone.

The outcome was surely unbefitting a home-grown commercial sector that had long dominated a worldwide market for
innovative medical devices. Furthermore, these events were a
particular embarrassment for acclaimed pioneer, Dow Corning,
whose achievements included major contributions to a wartime
victory and definition of the highest standards for an emerging
silicone product industry. When blame for the debacle was later
assigned, some were convinced that American enterprise was facing a breakdown in the integrity of its innovative process, while
others insisted the nation's regulatory procedures were both
flawed and entirely vulnerable to political influence.

Most interpreters were far too close to the controversy to
provide objective analysis. Yet when historical precedents were
considered, nobody should have been surprised by a conflict
between entrepreneurs and regulators. Since the days of Harvey
Washington Wiley and Asa Candler, when a fledgling Bureau of
Chemistry took on corporate giants like Coca-Cola, risk-taking
innovators have locked horns with regulators who are mandated
by the electorate to avoid risk.

Although the mammary implant was hardly a technological
match for more significant twentieth-century innovations such as

oral contraceptives and the transistor, its evolution was nonetheless representative of a long historical tradition for invention in
America. What had been demeaned as an "uninviting glue" by a
nineteenth century British chemist was in time rediscovered, not
in the United Kingdom or in Europe where chemical discovery was
a longstanding tradition, but in rural Corning, New York, where a
comparative novice gambled his career on a new approach to polymer synthesis. The results of his molecular maneuvering were
polymorphic compounds uniquely suited to the development of
myriad life-enhancing applications. Among the many marvels of
chemical ingenuity was a latticed matrix gel contained within an
elastomeric shell that attracted the attention of a visionary surgical
team searching for a synthetic facsimile of the female breast. After
refinements were made to the original design concept, clinical trials were conducted according to standards for that era.

Nothing was original about establishing the silicone medical product industry in quick time; its founding was based on the
same spirit of entrepreneurship that within a few decades doubled
mankind's life expectancy, reduced infant mortality by 90 percent,
halved the average work day, and produced more wealth than
had been created during the prior hundred thousand years. Yet,
none of the achievements that allowed mankind to work smarter
and live easier had come without taking risks, the kind of risks
that a society conceived in liberty had always been accustomed to
accepting.[388]

What then was so special about the silicone gel breast
implant that led to it becoming the catalyst for so much bureau-
cratic prejudgment, journalistic hyperbole, consumer angst,
generalized public rancor, professional frustration, and tort
opportunism?

To begin with, nearly all the risk analysis for mammary
devices was completed long before the FDA became responsible
for device oversight. Although safe limits for silicone tolerance
were defined in the 1940s and 1950s, this research was largely
disregarded by the agency, even though silicone polymers had
since become omnipresent in the environment. Never explained

by Commissioner Kessler or his staff was the basis for its focus on a single device while the food, beverage, and cosmetic industries—not to mention producers of several hundred more silicone devices—were never restricted from exposing the public to a polymer alleged to be toxic. It was not unreasonable to believe that Dr. Kessler's motive was more political than compassionate.

Silicone device manufacturers were ill-prepared for a review of their products that would systematically disregard decades of prior research, especially Dow Corning, whose products were developed in close collaboration with the medical profession. Manufacturers believed they had little to fear from a responsible product review. Instead, they faced the bizarre circumstance of a hearing room where the significance of past research was ignored while results from recently completed studies were declared inadmissible.

Plastic surgeons had convinced themselves that patient satisfaction rates exceeding 96 percent would surely carry the day, not an unreasonable position given sustained growth in demand for implants since 1962. Subsequent events proved them to be as wrong as the manufacturers were. Out of a population of hundreds of thousands, 4 percent who are less than fully satisfied can generate a tidal wave of discontent in the FDA's mailbox, and that is exactly what happened. And who could have anticipated that chance coincidental occurrence would produce the body of fear that resulted from concurrent threats of cancer and a portfolio of mysterious diseases? Yet similar behaviors are seen today in response to unfounded attacks on preservatives in vaccines, mercury in fish, amalgam in teeth, plastics in toys, and genetic modification of seeds.[389]

Legal scholar David Bernstein lists four requirements for what he terms phantom risk litigation: "first, actions of politically motivated individuals that downplay objective scientific inquiry; second, sensationalistic media coverage; third, public outrage at reports of corporate misconduct; and fourth, financial incentives that encourage attorneys and their clients to pursue claims built on dubious science." To this list can be added the political posturing of organizations, especially government agencies, with the power to select the evidence they wish to consider or ignore before they make policy decisions.

Senator Orrin Hatch, despite his prior sponsorship, was openly critical of David Kessler's service, particularly for his "self-serving behavior and his showboating." Hatch felt anger and regret "for the needless alarms given to countless women by the commissioner's handling of the breast implant affair." Charles Edwards, who ruefully acknowledged his role in recruiting Kessler, could not recall any prior commissioner hurting the agency as much by diverting resources away from so many more important issues. Former Deputy Commissioner Jim Benson, highly respected by his colleagues for always wanting to do the right thing and for deflecting unwarranted congressional invasions of proprietary data, later regretted the time wasted not only by the commissioner who wanted to read everything about breast implants—every letter and every PMA—but also by a staff who devoted twelve- and fourteen-hour days over the course of months and years. Asked if his boss had planned to shoot down breast implants, he said he didn't know but took note that every one of Kessler's moves played directly into the hands of trial lawyers. Benson understood that the manufacturers were not prepared to answer the many new questions and needed more time. He never understood the rush, wanted it all to be managed less visibly, but the commissioner always demanded full notice in the press.[390]

Was the FDA distracted from more important issues? Indeed it was. While the breast implant circus played out, Congress was deliberating a possible role for the FDA in regulating food supplements. In part because of too little input from a distracted agency, in part because of the long-standing record of an FDA dithering for years at a time over food innovations such as the sugar substitute cyclamate and the fat substitute Olestra, and in part because of uncommonly intense advocacy from one hundred million users of food supplements, we now have the Dietary Supplement Health and Education Act of 1994 (DSHEA) that excludes the FDA from regulatory oversight of more than five thousand unstudied substances. The same people fearful of chemicals in the environment enthusiastically consume unproven chemicals purchased at their local organic food superstores. Only in the event of measurable hazard can the agency act, as it finally did when Ephedra marketed by Metabolife was removed from the market, but not before more than one hundred reported deaths following its use.[391]

How do FDA actions stand up in court when challenged? Twenty-three federal cases were lost between 1990 and 2002, the judges questioning years of creative regulation writing, or ruling that the agency recklessly exceeded its authority. Perhaps most notable was the U. S. Supreme Court rejection of Dr. Kessler's attempt to regulate tobacco, noble in terms of smoking's lethal impact but naïve in terms of understanding the government's statutory limits. According to regulatory attorney and historian Peter Barton Hutt, "I don't know of any other time in history when the FDA has lost that many cases."[392]

But the problem is far greater than the folly of any single individual. Despite its immense power, the FDA is not capable of inventing anything; its decisions are based on information provided by the drug and device industry. While many of its professional staff have earned science degrees, very few are practicing scientists. Fewer still are experienced clinicians. Acquiring a science doctorate is one thing; conducting experiments, competing for grants, and publishing in peer-reviewed journals is quite another. This is not dereliction of duty but instead a feature of the FDA's present authority. Recognizing the difference between the functions of an investigator and the duties of a regulator helps to explain why the FDA was incapable of reordering the breast implant data to facilitate device approval as some believed it should have done.[393]

Dr. Henry Miller, who served under Kessler as director of the FDA's Office of Biotechnology, has recalled that the FDA he knew was largely made up of civil servants and political appointees, who felt constant pressure of scrutiny from Congress plus countless consumer watchdogs, all supported by a hostile press. Miller's Hoover Institution colleague and Nobel economist Milton

Friedman believed that an agency responsible for admitting or rejecting new products to the marketplace was vulnerable to making self-serving policy decisions. In so doing, it makes two kinds of errors. A Type 1 error is approving a harmful product; a Type 2 error is withholding a useful product. Postponing decisions altogether is the easiest course of all, as Dr. Kelsey learned when the thalidomide application sat on her desk for months without action.[394]

Comparisons with regulatory agencies abroad reveal how much longer the duration of clinical testing and regulatory scrutiny in the United States is. The European Medicines Agency (EMA) has been described as "lean, efficient, and remarkably well regarded by the drug industry." Unlike the FDA, the EMA maintains a close liaison with medical professionals and draws heavily from their considerable clinical expertise. The EMA is also perceived as client-friendly, relies heavily on summary reports supplied by product sponsors, and focuses its resources on drug safety. In contrast, the FDA treats drug and device companies like adversaries and functions more like a policing authority whose inspectors are permitted to carry small arms.[395]

As the end of President George H. W. Bush's term of office approached, word came from Secretary Sullivan's office that resignation letters were due. Dr. Kessler held out until he learned that President-elect Clinton planned to retain him. He served the FDA for two more years, during which time he devoted agency resources to a failed attempt at regulating tobacco. Meanwhile, the time required to bring a new drug to market, from synthesis to approval, increased to 14.8 years. (it had been 6.5 years in 1964). Costs of drug development reached five hundred million dollars, the highest price tag in the world (up 40 percent during Kessler's term).[396]

An incident reminiscent of circumstances leading to Dr. Wiley's 1912 resignation was reported by the *Associated Press* on Nov. 2, 1996. Dr. Kessler acknowledged careless handling of travel expense claims and wrote a check for an amount agreeable to the government. Soon after, he announced both his resignation and a plan to resume his career in academic administration as Dean of the Yale Medical School.[397]

In her 1996 book, *Science on Trial,* executive editor of the *New England Journal of Medicine* Marcia Angell disparages the anti-science bias seen among humanists, multiculturists, ecologists, and "alternative medicine" enthusiasts. She believes that science itself was on trial throughout the breast implant controversy and lost to the warped agendas of David Kessler and Sidney Wolfe, to an illusion of science offered by unqualified "experts," to reporters who prefer sensationalism wherever they can find it, and especially to the tort process that nurtures a jury's capacity to award millions based primarily on sympathy for the plaintiff. She urges a major reform of the tort system in three parts: 1) reduce incentives by eliminating contingency fees; 2) limit the use of juries in tort cases; 3) raise the standards for testimony heard from experts.[398]

In his *California Law Review* essay, David Bernstein considers each of these options in a broader legal context. The extremely unrealistic prospect of banishing contingency fees altogether does not preclude compromise choices such as "conditional fees," sometimes called "double or nothing" in the United Kingdom, where its use has successfully reduced speculative litigation yet continues to assure for ordinary citizens ready access to the courts.[399]

On limiting the role of juries in complex cases, the United States remains the only common law jurisdiction that has not yet abolished civil juries. Jurors like all people are by nature susceptible to emotion, and the clever trial lawyer has only to establish the prospect of evil intent, not difficult whenever the defendant is a large corporation. Alternatives to relying solely on a judge or a panel of judges include removal of damage award calculations from the hands of jurors, a revision that state court systems are beginning to establish.[400]

Bernstein documents ample precedent for raising standards of admissible expert testimony based on the Ninth Circuit Court of Appeals interpretation of *Daubert vs. Merrell Dow* (see previous chapter). Examples include the decisive action of Federal

District Judge Robert E. Jones, who appointed his own panel of experts and produced a dramatic turnaround in breast implant litigation not yet witnessed by Angell whose book preceded his action. Bernstein argues that given stricter standards of evidence, prior adoption of conditional fees, and established limitations on jury discretion, the breast implant litigation could not have evolved as it did. But such an occurrence, he adds, would leave other important questions unanswered, such as how best to deal with corporate misbehavior. Doesn't negligence that places the public's health at risk justify maintaining an approximation of the current tort system, he asks?

While *NEJM* Editor Angell is a more capable interpreter of the available scientific evidence than any attorney, was she, like Bernstein, justified in declaring that manufacturers were "negligent in their failing to undertake systematic studies of the health effects of breast implants?" With the intention of belaboring my point, I will list once again the following:

1. Silicone polymers were studied in 1948 by Dow Chemical toxicologists at the urging of Dow Corning and found to be uniquely well tolerated following injection, ingestion, and inhalation.
2. Silicones were studied in the laboratories of leading surgeons with support and encouragement from Dow Corning and all data reported promptly in respected journals.
3. The breast implant's impact on breast cancer, examined since 1974 with financial support from Dow Corning using epidemiologic methods, showed diminished incidence as of 1986. Five additional years of follow-up evidence corroborating previous findings was ruled inadmissible by the FDA in 1991.
4. Studies of gel bleed in capsules were conducted and reported in the 1970s by Rudolph and Abraham with financial support from McGhan Medical, documenting quantities of silicone visible only by electron microscopy without demonstrated clinical significance (consistent with Dow Corning measuring 0.1–0.5 grams of silicone migration per year).

5. Federally funded immuno-toxicology studies in the 1980s showed negligible silicone influence on immunity (referenced in 1991 Dow Corning PMA).
6. Early data from a cohort study by Weisman et al. and a case control study by Hochberg et al. showed normally expected rates of connective tissue diseases, all of this available to the FDA in several of the submitted PMAAs.
7. At request of McGann Medical Corporation, distinguished tumor biologist Gerhard Brand explained once more to the FDA why solid state carcinogenesis has nothing to do with the human condition. Johns Hopkins Professor of Immunology Noel Rose reminded the FDA that silicone polymers do not display adjuvant behavior in any reputable laboratory nor are there any validated reports of a human adjuvant disease.[401]

Does this sound like corporate misbehavior? Is it really a pack of errant manufacturers colluding to suppress a toxic reaction to breast implants? Or might the egregious behavior have been on the part of regulators, who were deliberately excluding critical evidence, evidence with a potential for reassuring many millions of people with silicone exposure? And to suggest that by the time of the hearings none of the manufacturers' data was credible is a lame excuse given the priority given to hit-and-miss anecdotes offered by activists and memoranda selected by trial attorneys for shock value alone. The scientific evidence listed above, every bit of it, was in Dr. Kessler's hands well in advance of his moratorium call, **and it all remains scientifically valid today**. More than two dozen additional studies of the autoimmune disease question confirm the earliest findings.

From a wide field of American producers of silicone medical products prior to the moratorium, there remained two survivors: Mentor Corporation (later Mentor Worldwide LLC) and Inamed (later Allergan). It took them six more years (1993–1999) to secure approval for saline-filled breast implants. Although Dr. Kessler had delegated responsibility for review of this category of devices to his deputy, Jane Haney (she later succeeded him as commissioner), nobody found the process to be any less frustrating. On January 8, 1993, the agency announced its call for safety and efficacy data pertaining to saline-filled breast implants. A sixty-day period was allowed for receipt of comments, a ritual that FDA staff were still not obligated to respond to. Hearings were held on June 2, 1993, and closed with a promise to reach a decision by year's end. But instead of its promised final decision, the FDA filed another of its "Talk Papers" on December 23, detailing additional studies it would require prior to approval, most of them dealing with the frequency of deflation and local complications. Not until November 12, 1999, did Mentor, and four days later Inamed, receive notice of saline implant approval for reconstruction and for augmentation beyond the age of 18.

In the midst of saline implant deliberations and without the traditional call for comments or hearings, the FDA approved a pilot study for women willing to receive breast implants filled with soybean oil instead of saline. It was an idea that for unexplained reasons Sidney Wolfe had taken a fancy to. Nine thousand pairs were sold in Europe impacting five thousand women. Following a brief period of availability in Belgium, they were banned from further use. Dreadful wounds resulted from continuous seepage of metabolic by-products of the decomposing fat passing through a permeable shell. Left unexplained was the sudden fascination and support for a device of this nature coming from steadfast critics of all breast implants. Had any of them taken into account that powerful immunologic adjuvants are commonly oil-based?[402]

As for the silicone gel breast implant, its trial would continue for another seven years. After traveling a torturous path that included submitting IDEs, conducting protocols, monitoring results, answering calls for data, reacting to deficiency notices, applying for approvals, testifying at hearings, gaining advisory panel support then losing it after panelists change their votes, receiving denials, resubmitting applications, responding to demands for additional studies, hearing rumors of preliminary approval, negotiating label requirements, and accepting limitations on product use, conditional approval came to both Mentor and Allergan in November 2006. But no one should have been surprised by any of this; the agency's glaring bias against the breast implant had been apparent since 1991. Yet throughout its fifteen years of review, the agency approved countless new and updated silicone devices while stubbornly adhering to the notion that just one silicone device in particular produced illness, perhaps even a mystery disease that had eluded medical science but not the FDA.[403]

When the silicone gel implant finally did receive full approval, the *Wall Street Journal* reported, "the facts finally overcame politics at the FDA." Public Citizen's Sidney Wolfe promptly labeled the gel implant "the most defective device ever approved by the FDA." NOW president Kim Gandy called it a "reckless decision." Yet approval did not come without conditions. In addition to the clinical data amassed for the 1991 PMAs and the mandated three- and four-year studies involving nearly fifty thousand patients, the agency required manufacturers to enroll another eighty thousand women and follow them for a decade. Implant recipients were advised to obtain frequent MRI examinations, which meant the cost of image surveillance might eventually exceed the original cost of surgery. And for what purpose? A failed implant is treatable with device replacement. Fortunately, this complication was becoming even less common because of stronger implant shells. And it remained to be seen how compliant patients would be when faced with these persisting invasions of privacy.[404]

Gathering in varied forums at various times since their interaction with the regulatory process, leaders of plastic surgery pondered the bruising experience and imagined how it might have transpired more favorably? How could the specialty more effectively react in the future? *Plastic and Reconstructive Surgery* Editor Robert Goldwyn was the gentle critic; he would have preferred that ASPRS take a more reflective approach. He blamed the PR firms for nurturing the fight. Yet he did not consider the breast implant crisis entirely bleak; "it made us better doctors." ASPRS Past President Elvin Zook held that plastic surgery's antagonistic reaction was misplaced and did not serve the specialty well, "and we were played for fools by the manufacturers." Past President James Hoehn observed that most ASPRS members had only rarely seen people as furious as the organized implant militants.

"Happy patients never form support groups," countered Norman Cole. "Only problem patients organize." Cole's wasn't the voice of a noncombatant; he had served as a combatant, facing down the breast implant's adversaries as ASPRS president during the 1991 hearings and the moratorium that followed. "As a [professional] society we were naïve in assuming that truth, science, and reason would decide the silicone crisis. This was decided by the politics of a special interest group because there was only one device targeted. After all, the medical profession could not function without silicone." For Cole there was nothing gentle or reflective about it. "I enjoyed the confrontations; I liked talking to Kessler eyeball to eyeball, conversing with Larry King. Yes, it was a lot of work but I did a credible job. And, of course, the facts were on our side."

"The relationship between physicians and manufacturers will be forever changed," added former PSEF President Fritz Barton. "Never again should medicine be willing to use a product from industry without being able to see the research data," momentarily overlooking the fact that his foundation's research committee was never denied information from any manufacturer, had never found any smoking guns, failed to discover any suppressed information of clinical significance. Yet there was considerable merit in his point; plastic surgeons needed to adopt means for evaluating devices intended for implantation independent of manufacturers. More specifically, successful implant surgery requires more systematic outcome measures than traditional case reporting.

Talk of avoiding another painful encounter with regulators led to visions of what appeared the ideal relationship maintained by the American Academy of Orthopedic Surgeons and the FDA. But their playing field is entirely different. Unlike breast implants, silicone devices for orthopedic problems are rarely challenged by the FDA. Regulators are less understanding of patients whose motive is to improve appearance. This was demonstrated once again during the agency's review of botulinum toxin A (Botox), a heat-killed extract previously approved for treatment of neuro-logical tics and idiopathic blepharospasm (involuntary blinking). Approval for treatment of facial wrinkles with Botox arrived years later and even then was soon attacked for labeling infractions. Allergan, its producer, had failed to specify exactly which wrinkle Botox was approved to treat.[405]

And if it was not enough for Americans to be confound-ed by risks they already faced in a society growing more complex by the day, another peril loomed: alleged conflicts of interest that challenged the integrity of an entire research community. Characterized by Harvard Professor of Medicine Thomas Stossel as a modern witch hunt, "a powerful anti-commercial advocacy movement threatens the momentum that brought us a windfall of new medical technologies, simply by imposing unrealistic restric-tions on physician/scientist participation." The very term "conflict of interest" implies wrongdoing. Instead of assuming scientists would want to protect their reputations, critics of industry assume the worst, believing that taking as little as a dollar from a drug or device company stands as proof of complicit dishonesty.[406]

Sidney Wolfe quickly jumped on this bandwagon, demand-ing that the FDA restrict from its advisory panels anyone with as much as a single link with industry. Public Citizen even object-ed to former NCI Director Andrew Eschenbach becoming acting FDA commissioner, the reason being that the government's best cancer specialists serve a duplicitous role when they advocate for new cancer drugs. Wolfe reviewed 221 panel meetings and dis-covered one-third of the participants had some prior tie with a medical product manufacturer; receiving an honorarium or a con-sulting fee was enough for guilt. Yet his own data failed to prove his point; commercial links made no impact on whether drugs or devices under review gained approval or not.[407]

Like witch hunts throughout history that spread more rap-idly than good sense can restrain, the search for criminal conflicts of interest now infects the appointment of federal grant reviewers and the publication of original work in scientific publications. *JAMA* not only insists that authors disclose industry support but also bans editorial commentary from anyone receiving compensation from industry. Yet the same tough-mindedness didn't apply to Public Citizen; readers were never told that the FDA adviser's financial connections failed to influence whether a product reached the marketplace.[408]

Often disregarded is the critical difference between "conflict" and "potential conflict" of interest. Everyone harbors a potential for conflict just as we all have moral standards we can abide by or abandon. For the 1992 hearing, announced conflicts ranged from the egregious—an ethicist without credentials providing testimony at a concurrent trial—to the nonexistent—surgeons arriving with the expertise and clinical experience they were selected by the agency to represent.

And so in America today, we have a highly empowered government agency, and dozens more like it, that in words close to those first offered by James Madison, "are enabled to control the governed, but [not yet] obliged to control themselves."[409]

EPILOGUE

Faced with uncertainty, best to do nothing.
—The Precautionary Principle

The collective mood of Dow Corning management and staff was suddenly lifted on the morning of June 1, 2004, by encouraging words from CEO Stephanie Burns. The company was finally emerging from nine long years of bankruptcy. Although Chapter 11 of the statutes governing corporation bankruptcy provides for temporary protection from creditors while a failing enterprise undergoes reorganization, Dow Corning never actually needed to reinvent itself. All it needed to get past was the threat of several thousand irate litigants, most of them recipients of breast implants, a product that never represented more than 1 percent of the company's revenue. Since 1995, when corporate attorneys filed for bankruptcy, Dow Corning continued to prosper as the world's largest producer of silicone polymers.[410]

Burns delighted in elaborating the company's financial position and its positive outlook for growth. Total sales revenue for the most recent quarter was up 20 percent to $713 million with the strongest performance coming from the electronics and semiconductor sectors. The bankruptcy hiatus had not distanced Dow Corning from the Internet revolution. Research and development continued at 6 percent of revenue and included imaginative projects like polycrystalline silicone wafers for chip production and light-emitting silicone diodes for high power/low energy light bulbs. Still in place from a prior corporate directive was Dow Corning's withdrawal from development, manufacture, and distribution of silicone products for plastic surgical implantation.

Nonetheless, Dow Corning continues to serve many other medical needs. Its silicone lubricants still coat most needles: hypodermic, suture, and acupuncture. Its elastomers remain in long-term implants such as hydrocephalus shunts and cardiac pacemakers. Dow Corning continues to serve as a health sciences innovator. Simethicone remains a component of antacid/antigas formulations.

Although operating income leaped 25 percent, net income fell 34 percent because of litigation costs, including a $30 million charge for Chapter 11 interest expense. Dow Corning's qualified claimants remain eligible for settlements ranging from two thousand dollars to two hundred and fifty thousand dollars without need to confirm any disease attributed to silicone, this despite over thirty studies showing no link between silicone exposure and autoimmune disorders or any other disease. This would seem to justify the observation dating from the seventeenth century that "the law is an ass." But there is more.[411]

Dow Corning recently experienced another adverse judicial ruling when an appellate court decided the two billion dollar fund established for implant claimants must be applied to tissue expanders if they were used in the breast region. The court was insensitive to Dow Corning's argument that tissue expanders are used for short periods to stimulate growth of skin. As of March 2014, the fund had paid $1.3 billion to one hundred and twenty-six thousand claimants, as much as three hundred thousand dollars for breast implant claims and as high as ten thousand dollars for related products such as hip and knee replacements, nose and chin implants, testicular and penile implants. A Dow Corning spokesman explained what should be obvious: enlarging the scope of claims necessarily leads to additional expenditures.[412]

While trial attorneys continued their efforts to collect every possible dollar from Dow Corning, several states were concerned about the adverse economic impact of tort litigation. Mississippi, Missouri, and Texas have enacted legislation that places a cap on noneconomic damages. They also put an end to "venue shopping," the practice of shifting cases into plaintiff-friendly jurisdictions regardless of where the alleged injury occurred. Efforts like these have reduced corporate exodus, attracted new business enterprise, and brought back doctors, especially obstetricians and neuro-surgeons, previously lost to prohibitive liability costs. Texas has experienced a 60 percent increase in medical license applications while a "loser pays" rule gains traction despite opposition from trial attorneys.[413]

At the federal level, there is little prospect for meaningful tort reform. Although the Supreme Court ruled in favor of Wal-Mart with respect to the basis for calculating class action punitive awards, it later held Wyeth Laboratories liable for failing to warn of side effects from a drug produced by another company. And any hope for malpractice liability reform implied by President Obama when he tried to enlist support from health professionals was lost to the complexities of the Affordable Care Act (ACA).[414]

America's present business unfriendly environment aside, medical device manufacturers continue to improve their products, although innovations are more likely seen first in Europe and Asia where research and clinical trials are more often conducted and where approvals are achieved faster. For example, a silicone polymer with greater cross-linkage of its units yields a more cohesive gel, assuring a more self-contained implant that holds its prescribed shape. Devices in Europe have benefited from these polymer innovations decades ahead of devices in the United States, where a change in polymer configuration can start the PMAA clock ticking all over again.

In Europe, the evaluation and approval of medical devices does not involve government regulators directly; instead there are third party "notified bodies" that test and certify according to recognized standards. Whereas a European device maker might achieve certification inside of a year or two, the most recent FDA review of a silicone gel breast implant required eleven years from initiation of a regulatory process. In 2012, Sientra, Inc. became the third American manufacturer, after Mentor and Allergan, permitted to market a full line of devices for cosmetic and recon-structive surgery.[415]

The American device industry is deeply concerned about a debilitating new tax written into the ACA. Instead of protect-ing a business sector that has long been a paragon of American inventiveness, legislators have imposed on device makers a 2.3 percent excise tax effective in 2013. What is especially pernicious about this tax is that it is levied on sales and not profits, meaning that after deducting costs, the tax can reduce profits by one-half or more. The most likely consequence will be tax "inversions," meaning cross-border mergers that remove tax obligations from IRS jurisdiction. Two years after the tax was announced, research and development spending fell from 6 percent to 2 percent in the U. S. but rose 22 percent in Southeast Asia. Vigorous efforts to repeal the tax are under way, but Congress has not acted.[416]

Never silent for long were the outspoken activists who con-tinued to believe that breast implants should be withheld from all women regardless of motive. They continued to hype platinum toxicity based on finding barely detectable amounts of platinate (the nontoxic salt of elemental platinum) in hair, nails, urine, and breast milk, all of this despite the Institute of Medicine's dismissal of all concerns about trace levels of minerals including platinum. Not yet acknowledged or likely to be was another encouraging epidemiologic study of breast cancer risk. There was sufficient follow-up (18.4 years) and enough implanted women enrolled (3,486) to establish statistical significance for a remarkable 26 percent reduction (53 cancers found; 72 expected).[417]

Renewed hope for genuine regulatory reform came in 2002 with the appointment of thirty-nine-year-old Mark McClellan, a medical doctor but also an economist and former member of President George W. Bush's Council of Economic Advisers. His appointment had been preceded by a twenty-two month leadership hiatus, the result of a diminishing field of "eligible" candidates; Senator Ted Kennedy, for example, announced he would block confirmation of anyone with prior ties to industry. A hiatus between FDA commissioners wasn't unusual. Since Dr. Kessler, the interregnum has averaged fifteen months. Looking back at the first twelve commissioners, the gap between them averaged two months.[418]

Like Dr. Kessler, Dr. McClellan arrived amid fanfare and brought with him a reputation for problem solving. Early measures included simplification of food labeling requirements: "Americans shouldn't need a science degree to figure out what foods fit into a healthy diet." He expanded the use of surrogate end points, laboratory or physical findings that predict drug efficacy, thereby reducing approval times by not having to demonstrate prolonged survival. December is the month with more product approvals than any other—assures a more impressive annual report—and this was especially true for McClellan's first year.[419]

But alas, McClellan would not be the regulatory miracle hoped for. After sixteen months of service, he was moved to manage Medicare. The FDA waited another sixteen months for the leadership of Lester M. Crawford, DVM, who lasted two months. Looking back on the McClellan term, former FDA Director Miller saw little evidence of genuine reform. In his view, the agency was largely staffed with people more interested in staying out of trouble than actually improving the public's health.[420]

As the agency's centennial observation approached, its history office was busily preparing celebratory posters with self-congratulatory themes: sulfanilamide, thalidomide, and the Dalkon Shield. But there were no festivals scheduled to celebrate efficiency. Development times and therefore development costs were increasing, according to the Tufts University Center for Drug Development. Direct and indirect costs of bringing new drugs to market now exceed one billion dollars, which explains why 80 percent of new drugs fail to recoup their development costs. How useful then are user fees paid by industry, $1.2 million per drug or device, enacted as an incentive to accelerate approvals?[421]

There is no shortage of inventive proposals for correcting the problems that plague the FDA, some of them coming from the agency's leadership, present and past. If the first part of solving a problem is admitting to it, the current commissioner, Margaret

Hamburg, did just that when she conceded, "the FDA is relying on 20th century regulatory science to evaluate 21st century medical products." Former Commissioner Eschenbach has argued passionately for accelerated approvals based on safety trials alone followed by postmarket monitoring of drug efficacy using the same study subjects. Former Biotechnology Director Miller cites proven advantages to the "Nationally Recognized Testing Laboratory" (NRTL) model. A ubiquitous and successful prototype is the nonprofit Underwriters Laboratories (UL), which tests and certifies twenty thousand categories of consumer products (some of them presenting hazards to life) at a fraction of the cost the FDA imposes. Miller discourages adoption of public-private development partnerships "to assure safe and effective drugs," as recently proposed by Maryland Senator Barbara Mikulski. The problem, he reminds us, is not scarcity of investment capital. Development resources are abundant. The problem is a bottleneck in the regulatory pipeline.[422]

In the aftermath of completing its hundredth year, the FDA courageously stood up to Public Citizen's charge that any celebration by the agency was nothing more than a fatuous propaganda campaign. Then it turned face and offered Sidney Wolfe a four-year term on its Drug Safety and Risk Management Committee. From that perch, he could more effectively challenge drugs and devices he considers superfluous ("Who needs it?"), thus limiting the competition that can reduce consumer prices. As the proud author of bestsellers *Pills That Don't Work,* and *Worst Pills: Best Pills,* he selectively attacks newer drugs still under patent in favor of older drugs, further driving up the costs of drug development.[423]

On a more positive note, plastic surgeons have actively pursued their dream of maintaining a more effective and credible interaction with the FDA. Expanding on the advisory committee format, both its trade group (ASPS) and its foundation (PSF) remain vigilant for problems involving the use of devices, seek advice from their own advisory panels, and on their own initiative forward information to the FDA. An excellent example involves the risk that never seems to go away, cancer following breast implantation.

Trial attorneys first called attention to "mysterious tumors" during the 1998 IOM review. At the time there was one published report of a lymphoma developing within the fibrous capsule surrounding a breast implant. Since then, seventy-seven such occurrences have been reported worldwide and another ninety-five unpublished cases found and surveyed. None are cancers of the breast gland itself but instead anaplastic large cell lymphomas (ALCL). Without a precise number of women with breast implants in hand (estimates range from twenty million to forty million) an incidence rate is not calculable. Estimates range from one in a half-million to one in a million. In other words rare. Despite attempts on the part of activists to attribute these tumors to silicone gel, they have also developed adjacent to saline-filled implants. Appearing to be specific to the texture-surface devices, they are thought to represent a manifestation of chronic inflammation.[424]

The question for this discussion is how are breast implant critics with historic bias (FDA) and enduring bias (Public Citizen) reacting to this news? Not unexpected is the fact that Dr. Wolfe has never retracted his "epidemic of breast cancer" prophecy, and if a tumor as rare as this one qualifies in his mind as an epidemic, then ALCL must represent a vindication for him. On his website, he accuses plastic surgeons of a cover-up based on a single careless remark instead of acknowledging the LA/USC team led by Drs. Brody and Deapen, whose devotion to monitoring cancer risk following breast implantation is now in its fortieth year. Wolfe lists thirty-four cases as his denominator so that he can exaggerate mortality risk. Nonetheless, deaths are a reality although not a certainty.[425]

The FDA response is a measured one unlike its reaction to sensational trial evidence in 1991. Its statement reads: "This should not be of major concern to patients as the absolute risk remains very low due to the extreme rarity of breast ALCL." As of this writing, the website acknowledges sixty cases identified via international regulatory agencies. Meanwhile there is effective continuing dialogue between plastic surgeons and the FDA.[426]

When ALCL and breast cancer are considered together, there might exist a risk-benefit tradeoff. If an implanted patient accepts a one in a half-million lymphoma risk, doesn't she also derive benefit from the observed reduction in breast cancer risk? The question is moot because women have never sought implants to avoid breast cancer; however, because some patients will refuse breast implants because of a remote chance of lymphoma, ALCL becomes a necessary part of informed consent.[427]

Soon after silicone gel breast devices received approval in 2006, requests for implantation reached three hundred thousand a year, according to ASPS surveys of plastic surgery procedures performed (manufacturers do not report sales in terms of device pairs sold). Demand for implants following the 1992 moratorium call had plunged 60 percent from one hundred and fifty thousand implanted during 1991. Remarkably, the 80:20 ratio of cosmetic to reconstructive procedures has remained constant. For patients with breast cancer treated by mastectomy, reconstruction rates as high as 70 percent are reported.[428]

Less fortunate are the women who suffer genuine rheumatic illness and are still led to believe their symptoms evolve from silicone exposure. Not even thirty consecutive studies that disprove a causal link, nor thirty more, are likely to change their convictions. But as former president John Adams once observed, "Facts are stubborn things, and whatever may be our wishes, our inclinations, or the dictates of our passions, they cannot alter the state of facts and evidence." While I can hope this book might provide comfort for all prior implant recipients, I am more likely to inform and thus reassure those who seek implantable silicone devices for the first time.[429]

Every prospective patient knows why she pursues breast implant surgery; few others can even begin to understand, and too many are quick to judge. Some insist on imposing their will on others. Naysayers aside, because of its inherent molecular structure, silicone remains as biocompatible as it was initially found to be. The diversity of current applications in industrial, electronic, and

Before	After

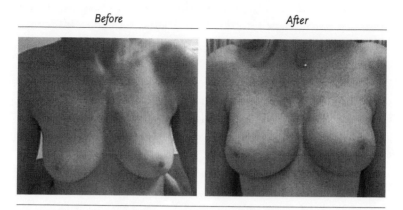

39 yr. old mother of three with lobular breast carcinoma; bilateral nipple sparing mastectomies with immediate reconstruction using expanders and then implants. This patient did not have to experience mastectomy defects.
CREDIT: Anne Wallace MD

medical fields exceeds the wildest imaginations of the polymer's original pioneers. But prospective beneficiaries of silicone devices now live in a society where the precautionary principle prevails: *when faced with uncertain consequences, the best course is to avoid taking action.*[430]

Also referred to as the "paralyzing principle," it is no principle at all; instead, it is a plausible-sounding excuse for opposing innovation. Neither is precautionary inertia a sustainable force, or there would be little progress at all. Yet we still have at our disposal the traditional aphorisms advancing its popularity: "better safe than sorry," "an ounce of prevention is worth a pound of cure," "look before you leap," "if it saves just one more life," and from Hippocrates himself, "first, do no harm."

There is nothing wrong with caution in the face of authentic danger or an unfavorable risk-benefit relationship, but when we apply the precautionary principle to remote hazards, or worse, to hypothetical perils, we leave the world of science and enter the realm of ideology. We fall under the spell of those who covet a return to some imagined preindustrial back-to-nature idyll, and we distract ourselves from genuine risks and calamities. Should we focus our efforts on the songbirds (who never actually succumbed to DDT) or on persisting deaths from mosquito-borne diseases that number in the millions?[431]

The impossibility of eliminating all risks should be obvious to all. How best then to break free of the precautionary principle's grip on society and its appointed government regulators? This cannot happen without major progress in math and science literacy. For example, until there is greater familiarity with quantitative measures such as relative risk, especially by those who report science in the popular media, Americans will remain susceptible to false fears based on false science or false interpretations of science, just as so many were when Dr. Wiley's infant bureau of chemistry began its relentless quest for power more than a century ago.

GLOSSARY OF ACRONYMS

AAJ	American Association for Justice (since 2006)
ACA	Affordable Care Act
ALCL	Anaplastic Large Cell Lymphoma
AP	*Associated Press*
ASAPS	American Society for Aesthetic Plastic Surgery
ASPRS	American Society of Plastic and Reconstructive Surgeons
ASPS	American Society of Plastic Surgeons (since 1998)
ATLA	Association of Trial Lawyers of America
BFDI	Board of Food and Drug Inspection
CDRH	Center for Devices and Radiologic Health (FDA)
CTN	Command Trust Network
DCC	Dow Corning Corporation
DCW	Dow Corning Wright
DHEW	Department of Health, Education, Welfare
DHHS	Department of Health and Human Services
DSHEA	Dietary Supplement Health & Education Act
EMA	European Medicines Agency
FDA	Food and Drug Administration
FDR	Franklin Delano Roosevelt
FTC	Federal Trade Commission
GRAS	Generally Regarded as Safe
HHS	Health and Human Services
IDA	Investigational Drug (Device) Application
IDE	Investigational Device Exemption
IND	Investigational New Drug
IOM	Institute of Medicine
IUD	Intra-uterine Device
JAMA	*Journal of the American Medical Association*

LA/USC	Los Angeles/University of Southern California (cancer study)
MDR	Medical Device Reporting (FDA)
MTD	Maximum Tolerated Dose
NAS	National Academy of Sciences
NCI	National Cancer Institute
NDA	New Drug Application
NEJM	*New England Journal of Medicine*
NIH	National Institutes of Health
NRTL	Nationally Recognized Testing Laboratories
NYT	*New York Times*
PID	Product Information Document
PRS	*Plastic and Reconstructive Surgery*
PSEF	Plastic Surgery Educational Foundation
PSF	Plastic Surgery Foundation (since 2011)
PMA(A)	Pre-Market Approval (Application)
SEER	Surveillance, Epidemiology, End Results Program (NCI)
SIRC	Silicone Implant Research Committee (PSEF)
TR	Theodore Roosevelt
UL	Underwriter Laboratories
USDA	United States Department of Agriculture
USDHHS	United States Department of Health and Human Services
WSJ	*Wall Street Journal*

CHRONOLOGY

1824   Jons Jakob Berzelius, Swedish Chemist, discovers the element silicon.

1862   President Lincoln appoints a chemist, Charles Weatherill, to serve in the Department of Agriculture's new Bureau of Chemistry, forerunner of today's Food and Drug Administration.

1883   Dr. Harvey Washington Wiley is appointed chemist, USDA Bureau of Chemistry, by Secretary of Agriculture George Loring.

1897   Frederick Stanley Kipping (1863–1949) is elected a Fellow of the Royal Society and appointed Professor of Chemistry, University College Nottingham. A pioneer in the study of organosilicons, he coins the term silicone from two established chemical terms, silicon and ketone.

1902   Biologics Control Act passed to ensure purity and safety of serums and vaccines used to prevent diseases.

1906   On June 30, Theodore Roosevelt signs into law both the Meat Inspection Act and the Pure Food and Drugs Act of 1906. Later he lists these among his major presidential achievements.

1909   Dr. Wiley orders seizure of forty barrels and twenty kegs of Coca-Cola syrup in Chattanooga, Tennessee.

1909   Biologist Clarence Little begins experiments that will yield strains of inbred (virtually identical) mice, later shown to be of sufficient genetic weakness to become tumor-prone. Establishes Jackson Laboratory in 1929.

1911   *United States vs. Forty Barrels and Twenty Kegs of Coca-Cola:* A US District Court judge finds the defendant innocent of charges of adulteration and misbranding. A US Appellate

Court later upholds the verdict. The Supreme Court later remands (returns) the case, reestablishing the law's jurisdiction over products regardless of formulation or trademark.

1914 *United States vs. Lexington Mill and Elevator:* Supreme Court rules that the government must show a relationship between a chemical additive and the alleged harm it causes in humans.

1927 Bureau of Chemistry reorganized as Food, Drug, and Insecticide Administration. Three years later, it becomes the Food and Drug Administration.

1933 First bill is introduced to revise the 1906 Food and Drugs Act now considered obsolete, launching a five-year legislative battle.

1937 Elixir Sulfanilamide Massengill kills 107 in Tulsa, Oklahoma.

1938 FDR signs into law the Federal Food, Drug, and Cosmetic Act of 1938 requiring new drugs to be shown safe prior to marketing, authorizing factory inspections, adding the power of imposing court injunctions.

1940 Naval liaison officer (later Admiral) Hyman Rickover places an order for 990A resin, the first commercial silicone product developed by Corning Glass chemist J. Franklin Hyde.

1943 Corning Glass and Dow Chemical establish a joint venture, Dow Corning Company of Midland, Michigan.

1944 First biomedical application of polydimethylsiloxane is lubrication of syringes used to administer earliest doses of "miracle drug," penicillin.

1946 The Federal Administration Act of 1946 hands more power to all branches of government, empowering them to establish regulations independent of legislative action, albeit answerable to subsequent legal challenge.

1958 Dow Corning establishes The Center for Aid to Medical Research.

1958 Delaney Clause added to the Food Additive Amendment restricting use of any substance found to cause cancer in any animal species (ignores fact that mouse strains used for testing are by genetic definition tumor prone).

1961 Potential use of a Dow Corning silicone product for breast surgery explored by Drs. Thomas Cronin and Frank Gerow of Houston, Texas.

1962 Houston patient Timmie Jean Lindsay receives first silicone gel mammary devices for cosmetic breast enlargement.

1964 Dow Corning announces establishment of its Silicone Injection Committee listing nine surgeon consultants; files with FDA for an Investigational New Drug exemption.

1974 Drs. Garry Brody and Dennis Deapen inaugurate Los Angeles/USC cohort study of breast cancer risk among women with breast implants.

1976 Medical Device Amendments passed to ensure safety and effectiveness of medical devices including diagnostic products.

1976 General and Plastic Surgery Devices Advisory Panel recommends that silicone gel-filled breast implants remain classified as Class II (performance standards required).

1978 Drs. Rudolph and Abraham establish method for detecting silicone gel bleed in capsule; find no correlation between contraction and bleed.

1977 Houston attorney Robert Mithoff wins $170,000 award for Cleveland woman (*Corley vs. Dow Corning*) claiming rupture, pain, and suffering.

1982 FDA proposes placing all breast implants in Class III, requiring stricter controls. Plastic surgeons through their trade organization, ASPRS, join device manufacturers in protest of this decision.

1984 *Stern vs. Dow Corning*: $1.7M award, $1.5M of which is punitive.

1986 First reading of data from LA/USC study reveals slightly lower risk of breast cancer among women with breast implants.

1988 (June 24) FDA publishes rule assigning breast implants to Class III requiring submission of premarket approval applications (PMA).

1988 (November 2) Dow Corning reveals results of rodent

experiments showing tumors consistent with solid state carcinogenesis first described in 1941.

1988 (November 9) Sidney Wolfe of Public Citizen, presumably shown data by an FDA staffer, makes findings public, predicts a breast cancer epidemic among women with breast implants and demands that FDA ban the device.

1988 (November 22) FDA Commissioner Frank Young writes Sidney Wolfe citing consultation with cancer authorities, who determine reported tumors to be a rodent-specific phenomenon without need for banning silicone devices.

1988 (November 22) Meeting of General and Plastic Surgery Device Advisory Panel at which Sidney Wolfe, Sybil Goldrich testified, as well as Dan Bolton, who violates a judge's gag order and reveals content of selected Dow Corning documents used as evidence in *Stern vs. Dow Corning* trial.

1990 (December 10) *Face to Face with Connie Chung* sends a shockwave of fear to viewers, all based on four anecdotes and selected commentary from "experts" later disqualified from testifying in American courtrooms.

1990 (December 18) Representative Ted Weiss convenes Subcommittee on Human Resources and Intergovernmental Relations for a hearing titled, "The Dangers of Silicone Breast Implants: Is the FDA Protecting Patients?"

1991 Several state legislatures—California, Texas, and Maryland among them—pass bills mandating patient information summaries for breast implants.

1991 (April) FDA publishes final rule setting deadline for manufacturer submission of PMAs within ninety days.

1991 (April 14–25) Over a span of eleven days, NYT quotes anonymous FDA source predicting deaths from polyurethane breast implants at two hundred to four hundred a year, followed by ABC-TV citing a 1:10,000 cancer risk, followed by an FDA "talking paper" announcing risk is too small to warrant implant removal, followed by FDA "backgrounder" citing a woman's lifetime risk of cancer from polyurethane implants at one in a million.

1991 (July) Dow Corning and other manufacturers deliver nine PMAs to FDA.

1991 (September) FDA declares all submitted PMAs to be unsatisfactory; informs *New York Times* before notifying manufacturers.

1991 (November) Despite data omissions, General and Plastic Surgery Devices Advisory Panel votes unanimously to recommend continued availability of breast implants to fill a public need for reconstruction following cancer.

1991 (December) *Hopkins vs. Dow Corning* : $7.3 million award, $6.5 million is punitive.

1992 (January) FDA Commissioner David Kessler asks for a voluntary moratorium on continued use of silicone gel breast implants, ignoring advisory panel recommendation. Worldwide reaction follows.

1992 (February) Advisory Panel meets again to consider new evidence of diseases; hears from two rheumatology consultants who doubt existence of link. Manufacturers restricted from presenting new data since 1991 PMA.

1992 (March) Dow Corning withdraws from plastic surgery device market but continues as a major supplier of silicone polymers and health products.

1992 Moratorium reversed; gel implants limited to breast reconstruction conducted under approved protocol limitations imposed by FDA.

1992 (December) *Johnson vs. Bristol-Myers Squibb*: $25 million award, $20 million punitive.

1993 (January 8) FDA calls for safety and effectiveness data for saline-filled implants, setting a sixty-day period for receipt of comments.

1994 (June 2) FDA conducts hearing on saline-filled implants; promises decision by end of year.

1994 (December) Instead of the promised decision, FDA issues a "Talk Paper" detailing the additional studies it will require before approving saline-filled breast implants.

1994 (July) FDA grants conditional approval for pilot study of a

breast implant filled with so-called "purified soybean oil."
See text for tragic outcome.

1995 (May) Dow Corning files for Chapter 11 bankruptcy protection, halting more than 20,000 lawsuits and 400,000
claims against global settlement.

1999 Mentor (November 12) and Inamed (formerly McGhan)
(November 16) receive their approvals for marketing saline-
filled implants for reconstruction and for augmentation of
patients over eighteen.

2000 (August) FDA approves Mentor's IDE for study of silicone
gel breast implants at a limited number of sites.

2002 (December) Inamed applies for approval to market silicone
gel breast implants.

2003 (October) FDA panel recommends approval of Inamed's
application but with conditions.

2003 (December) Mentor applies for approval to market silicone
gel breast implants.

2005 (April) An FDA panel recommends denial of an updated
application by Inamed that was approved at an earlier panel
meeting but recommends approval of an application by
Mentor with conditions.

2005 (July) Mentor and (September) Inamed receive preliminary
notice of pending approval.

2006 (November) FDA issues final approvals to both Mentor and
Allergan (formerly Inamed) for silicone gel breast implants,
fifteen years and four months after issuing call for PMAAs.

2012 (March) FDA notifies Sientra of approval for its gel implant,
making it the third American supplier since 1992 permitted to market a full line of devices for cosmetic and
reconstructive breast surgery.

SOURCE NOTES

Prologue

1   Sandra Blakeslee, "Unapproved Breast Implant Seized," *New York Times,* July 30, 1991. Additional details of the seizure are based on eyewitness accounts reported to the company's board of directors and interviews with Robert Ersek, an officer of Bioplasty.

2   FDA Commissioner Kessler's statement was released by the Minneapolis field office of the FDA at the time of the seizure, reported in Twin City newspapers, and quoted during local television coverage of the incident. For Bioplasty's mammography claim, see A. A. Beisang, R. A. Geise, R. A. Ersek, "A Radiolucent Prosthetic Gel" *Plastic and Reconstructive Surgery,* 87 (May 1991) 855–92.

3   Bioplasty Inc. filed for relief under Chapter 11 of Title 11, U.S Code on April 29, 1993. Meanwhile, devices of similar content remained marketable without restriction in Europe.

4   Dr. Kessler on January 6, 1992, called for a voluntary moratorium on use of silicone gel breast implants. The worldwide reaction to this action is described in Chapter 12.

5   In time, statements were issued by the American Medical Association, American College of Surgeons, American Cancer Society, American College of Radiology, American College of Rheumatology, American Society of Clinical Oncology, American College of Pathology, and many more professional groups. Dr. Kessler made his often-quoted reference to tires in a statement issued from Rockville, MD, on April 16, 1992, nearly three months after his moratorium call.

6   Numerous descriptions of the Chattanooga seizure appear in the historiography of the Coca-Cola Corporation and

among the personal recollections of Harvey Washington Wiley. I have relied on two recent comprehensive histories of Coca-Cola: Frederick Allen, *Secret Formula* (New York: Harper Collins, 1994) and Mark Pendergrast, *For God, Country, and Coca-Cola* (New York: Macmillan, 1993). Dr. Wiley provided his version of the event in his autobiography: *H. W. Wiley: Autobiography* (Indianapolis: Bobbs-Merrill, 1930). "Dope," a term deplored by Asa Candler, became a popular slang term for Coca-Cola before "Coke" replaced it.

7   See US vs. Forty Barrels and Twenty Kegs of Coca Cola. *Federal Reporter* 191 (1911): 431–40, for outcome of Chattanooga trial.

8   Historians of Wiley's influence on the food law often rely on his autobiography. Wiley is remarkably consistent, even reporting in detail the public's critical reaction to his convictions, yet always pointing out how wrong they were. For David Kessler's education and career, see his own personal recollections in *A Question of Intent: A Great American Battle with a Deadly Industry* (New York: Public Affairs/Perseus Books Group, 2001), 3–17.

9   Throughout Dr. Wiley's public oratory and writing, he expresses concern for the public's welfare. Dr. Kessler made his case for restriction of silicone breast implants in the *New England Journal of Medicine:* "The Basis for the FDA's Decision on Breast Implants" *NEJM,* 326 (1992): 1713–15. For a critique of David Kessler, see Marcia Angell, who was executive editor of the *New England Journal of Medicine* at the time of the controversy, published her interpretation of the controversy and its legal consequences in *Science on Trial* (New York: W. W. Norton, 1996).

10   Although the committee underwent changes of name, I refer to its first appellation, Silicone Implant Research Committee (SIRC) of the PSEF. Ever since its inception, the committee held that the issue was not limited to breast implants. If silicone proved to be toxic, the danger would necessarily apply to all silicone devices. DISCLOSURE:

Following my chairmanship of SIRC, I agreed to support defendants or plaintiffs involved in legal actions, but only if my testimony was limited to the scientific evidence pertaining to medical and surgical uses of silicone polymers.

11   Dr. Wolfe's timing could not have been better. His announcement coincided with the annual meeting of the American College of Surgeons, a week when the media traditionally reports advances in the surgical sciences.

12   Mariann Hopkins v. Dow Corning Corporation. $7.3 million awarded by jury on December 13, 1991.

13   The author's observations are recalled from attendance of FDA hearings in Baltimore, Bethesda, and Gaithersburg, MD, during 1991 and 1992. The *New York Times* reporter was Philip J. Hilts.

14   The author was one of several waiting to query Dr. Wolfe following his public remarks, but he refused us, claiming a very tight schedule, and then turned to reporters awaiting him.

15   ASPRS President William Porterfield filed a petition urging the FDA to assign the silicone gel breast implant to its Class II, hoping to avoid the necessity of a full review.

16   Robert Rylee explained to plastic surgeons the importance of maintaining privacy of proprietary data; rheumatologist Thomas Sergent predicted that incentives for claiming rheumatic illness after breast implantation would invalidate future epidemiologic studies.

17   Earl L. Warrick, *Forty Years of Firsts: The Recollections of a Dow Corning Pioneer* (New York: McGraw-Hill, 1990).

18   The author, like most plastic surgeons in America, recalls hundreds of conversations with patients alarmed by the reports appearing in their newspapers on their television screens. Most wanted reassurance; only a few wanted their implants removed.

19   Statement of Congresswoman Marilyn Lloyd before the General and Plastic Surgery Device Advisory Panel, February 19, 1992.

Chapter 1

20   Thomas Jefferson, *Notes on Virginia*, Query XVII, (1781–1785).

21   News of "Dr. Wiley's Resignation" appeared as an editorial in *Scientific American*, March 30, 1912, 282. Its author condemned the unscientific workings of the Bureau of Chemistry under Wiley. The Augean Stables of mythology housed 3,000 oxen and had not been cleaned in thirty years. In Wiley, *Autobiography*, the author delights in his staff labeling him a "zealot."

22   Wiley acknowledges his unwillingness to revise an established position in the face of new scientific evidence in Wiley, *Autobiography*, 116–22. Refer also to Clayton Coppin and Jack High, *Politics of Purity: Harvey Washington Wiley and the Origins of Federal Food Policy* (Ann Arbor: University of Michigan Press, 1999). See Peter Barton Hutt, "The Transformation of United States Food and Drug Law," *Journal of the Association of Food & Drug Officials:* 60 (1996): 1–62.

23   Wiley, *Autobiography*, 1–40.

24   Suzanne White Junod, "Harvey Wiley: His Life and Times," *The Food and Drug Law Institute Update*, June 2000 (http://www.fdli.org). Also refer to James Harvey Young, "Three Southern Food and Drug Cases" *Journal of Southern History* 49 (February 1983): 3–36. Alum refers to salts of aluminum whereas saltpeter is potassium nitrate, a naturally occurring salt used in gunpowder.

25   Ibid., 98–112.

26   Wiley, *Autobiography*, 138–49. Corn sugar provides half the sweetness of sucrose at a fraction of the cost. Why Wiley had a problem with corn-derived sugar is not clear.

27   James Harvey Young, *Pure Food: Securing the Federal Food and Drugs Act of 1906* (Princeton, NJ: Princeton University Press, 1989). See also Daniel Boorstin, *The Americans: The Democratic Experience* (New York: Vintage Books, 1973), 309–31, for a discussion of advances in food processing.

28   Wiley's technology was based on refraction, a physical prop-
      erty of a sugar's ability to rotate a beam of light. Dextrose
      is named for rotating to the right (dextra is Latin for right).
      Wiley's apparatus was a primitive version of a refractometer,
      later replaced by light spectrophotometry, a standard tech-
      nology for analytical chemical testing today.

29   That Wiley enjoyed telling this story is apparent from the
      fact that it appears often in his writing. See Wiley, *Autobiog-
      raphy,* 150–62.

30   When Wiley returned to Purdue in 1921 to deliver a com-
      mencement address, he visited the university's museum
      and saw his notoriously conspicuous nickel-plated bicycle
      on display there.

31   H. W. Wiley, *History of a Crime Against the Food Law,* 1929.
      This is a self-published polemic citing his personal griev-
      ances against all those who opposed him throughout his
      career.

32   Wine has long been sweetened with sucrose as well as dex-
      trose. Wiley attacked only what he considered the "deceptive"
      addition of dextrose to wine. In France, it is unlawful to add
      any sugar to wine to boost alcohol and thus cover for imma-
      ture grapes.

33   Felipe Fernandez-Armesto, *Near a Thousand Tables: A His-
      tory of Food,* (New York: The Free Press, 2002), 187–224.
      For dairy industry testimony before Congress, see H.R. Rep.
      No. 1529, 47th Congress., 1st Sess. 3 (1882). Young, in *Pure
      Food: Securing the Federal Food Drugs Act of 1906,* discusses
      the oleomargarine controversy, highlights Dr. Wiley's lim-
      ited role but does not indicate whether Wiley was simply
      deferring to the dairy industry's critical stand or if oleomar-
      garine lay beyond his own perceived responsibility.

34   Notes and letters found in Wiley's papers, Manuscript Divi-
      sion, Library of Congress.

35   Born in Scotland in 1835 and raised in Iowa, Wilson farmed
      before pursuing a political career. Wilson's government
      service from 1897 to 1913 is documented in an obituary

published by the *Chicago Tribune* on August 25, 1921. After resigning, he became a professor of agriculture at Iowa State University in Ames, Iowa.

36   Gunther W. Plaut, *The Torah: A Modern Commentary* (New York: Union of American Hebrew Congregations, 1981), 808–13. Food laws in early civilizations are also documented by Peter Barton Hutt in "A History of Government Regulation of Adulteration and Misbranding of Food," *Food, Drug, Cosmetic Law Journal* 39 (1984), 2–5.

37   Lemuel Shattuck, *Report of the Sanitary Commission of Massachusetts*, 1850, 28–48 as cited by Hutt, "A History of Government Regulation of Adulteration and Misbranding of Food," 45. Readers surprised by the data need remember that life expectancy is not the same as life span. The reported mean is reduced by infant mortality from contagious diseases prevalent in that day.

38   Felipe Fernandez-Armesto, *Near a Thousand Tables: A History of Food,* (New York: The Free Press, 2002), 44–45.

39   Numerous histories of the "Poison Squad" are available. Refer to Young's *Pure Food*, 151–56, and Coppin and High's *The Politics of Purity,* for an interpretation that highlights the folly of Wiley's misguided attempt to conduct valid scientific experiments.

40   The term "poison squad" was coined by George Rothwell Brown, a young reporter for the *Washington Post,* who began writing about the experiments in 1902 and made it his pet journalistic endeavor for as long as the studies continued.

41   See Young, *Pure Food*, 156–57.

42   James Harvey Young, "Two Hoosiers and the Two Food Laws of 1906." *Indiana Magazine of History* 88 (1992): 303–19.

43   Claims of deaths in the hundreds appearing in Fernandez-Armesto's *Near a Thousand Tables: A History of Food,* 187–224 were not reported at the time. Noncombatant deaths from contagion were commonplace as in all prior wars, but no mortality from canned meat is recorded.

44   A sampling is offered here for readers curious about what
      Sinclair observed: "There was never the least attention paid
      to what was cut up for sausage; there would come all the way
      back from Europe old sausage that had been rejected, and
      that was moldy and white—it would be dosed with borax
      and glycerine, and dumped into the hoppers and made over
      again for home consumption. There would be meat that
      had tumbled out on the floor, in the dirt and sawdust, where
      the workers had tramped and spit uncounted consumption
      germs. There would be meat stored in great piles in rooms;
      and thousands of rats would race about on it. These rats
      were nuisances and the packers would put out poisoned
      bread for them; they would die and then rats, bread, poison,
      and meat would all go into the hoppers together."

45   Beveridge to Albert Shaw, May 26, 1906, Beveridge Papers,
      Manuscript Division, Library of Congress, cited by Young,
      "Two Hoosiers and the Two Food Laws of 1906, 315.

46   Ibid., 318. Also, for interpretation of inertia characteristic
      of the U. S. Senate during what has been called the Gilded
      Age of America, see Robert Caro, *The Years of Lyndon John-
      son: Master of the Senate* (New York: Alfred Knopf, 2002),
      33–35.

47   Ironically, Upton Sinclair was unhappy with the Meat
      Inspection Act because it did nothing for the men who
      toiled in the abattoirs: "As for the men who worked in tank-
      rooms full of steam, in some of which there were open vats
      near the level of the floor, their peculiar trouble was that
      they fell into the vats; and when they were fished out, there
      was never enough of them left to be worth exhibiting . . .
      until all but the bones of them had gone out to the world as
      Durham's Pure Lard!" Later he famously declared, "I aimed
      at the public's heart and by accident hit it in the stomach."
      Cited by Kolko, *Triumph of Conservatism*, 103, 107.

48   See Wiley, *Autobiography*, 241, for a detailed exchange with
      the president. Also see Young, *Pure Food*, 271–72, for corre-
      spondence describing the pen incident.

49   Wiley, *Autobiography,* 238.

50   National Archives II in Beltsville, MD, holds several boxes of index cards pleading for seizure of food shipments believed to be in violation of the 1906 law. Three requests to seize Coca-Cola syrup in 1909 were denied but a fourth was approved, a decision that in time produced a stronger law.

51   Charles Howard Candler, *Asa Griggs Candler* (Atlanta: Emory University Press,1950), 63–65.

52   Ibid. See also Pendergrast, *For God, Country, and Coca-Cola,* and Allen, *Secret Formula,* provides documentation of Pemberton's nerve tonics and the particular concoction that became a popular soft drink.

53   Charles Howard Candler, "The True Origins of Coca-Cola," Coca-Cola Miscellany: Special Collections, Woodruff Library, Emory University.

54   U. S. Circuit Court, Northern District of Georgia, Feb. 2, 1902. The Internal Revenue Service was ordered to return to the Coça-Çola Company the tax that had been paid under protest, a sum of $10,858.76 plus all accrued interest.

55   Candler, "The True Origins of Coca-Cola," 10. In a letter to Wiley, Candler declared that Coca-Cola was no more to blame for putting caffeine in its beverage than the US government could be condemned for importing tea and coffee. But Wiley distinguished between a poison that is present in a natural product and one that is added to an artificial one. "You might as well say that hydrocyanic acid is harmless," he said, "because it occurs in peaches and almonds."

56   Process for removing residual cocaine subcontracted by Coca-Cola to Maywood Chemical Company in New Jersey.

57   Wiley comments sparingly on the trial in his *Autobiography* but offers considerable detail about his difficulty interacting with Wilson during much of his tenure as chief chemist.

58   Ludy T. Benjamin, Anne M. Rogers, Angela Rosenbaum, "Coca-Cola, Caffeine, and Mental Deficiency: Harry Hollingworth and the Chattanooga Trial of 1911," *Journal of the History of Behavioral Sciences,* 27 (1991): 42–55.

59 These are typical agreements made by universities and other nonprofit research institutions before accepting research support from corporations or other private entities. The institution usually secures the right to publish the results regardless of the findings.

60 Cited in Benjamin et al., "Coca-Cola, Caffeine," footnote No. 7.

61 Hollingworth's data was later used in a scientific publication that stands as a classic work on the effects of caffeine on cognition, as well as a model for conducting clinical trials. See H. L. Hollingworth, "The Influence of Caffein on Mental and Motor Efficiency," *Archives of Psychology* 22 (1912): iii.

62 Today, this experimental design is called a crossover study. A subject begins in one experimental group and later crosses over to another group.

63 Philip Mooney, Coca-Cola Corporation archivist, provided copies of the *Chattanooga News* coverage that were clipped and distributed following the trial as a marketing exercise. Concerned that the articles might have been selected for the corporate viewpoint, I have compared testimony reported in the *News* with testimony selected by the respective judges. Today, reporters rarely record testimony in similar detail because of court reporters; expert witnesses today are not allowed to hear prior expert testimony.

64 *Chattanooga News*, March 10, 1909.

65 See Benjamin's "Coca-Cola, Caffeine," 48–49. Also, Professor Hollingworth reflected on his court testimony in an unpublished autobiography titled, *Years at Columbia*. Failing to define the financial relationship between an expert and the corporation he/she is testifying for would be considered malpractice in a contemporary tort action.

66 Judge Sanford's decision dealt only with questions of law, meaning the Pure Food Act's jurisdiction over allegations filed by the Bureau of Chemistry. Without a jury verdict, the important question of fact, whether or not caffeine was poisonous to humans, was not determined.

67   Wiley, *History of a Crime Against the Food Law*, 887 (Wiley provides transcription of actual testimony given before the Moss Committee).

68   "Dr. Wiley's Resignation," *Scientific American*, March 12, 1912, 282.

69   Wiley, *Autobiography*, 248.

70   Letter from Peter Hutt to author, March 31, 2003.

71   Mary W. M. Hargreaves, "The Durum Wheat Controversy," in *Agricultural History*, 42 (1968) 211–29. *Lexington Mill & Elevator Co. vs. United States* 202 Fed. 615, District Court of Appeals, Eighth Circuit, Jan. 23, 1913.

Chapter 2

72   See Earl L. Warrick, *Forty Years of Firsts: Recollections of a Dow Corning Pioneer* (New York: McGraw-Hill, 1990), 106, for reference to this comment first expressed by Kipping prior to the 1907 publication of his findings: *Journal of the Chemical Society*, 91 (1907): 209.

73   Warrick, *Forty Years of Firsts*, 21. Rickover, later Admiral Rickover, distinguished himself as a nuclear submarine pioneer.

74   For additional biographical detail see Warrick, *Forty Years of Firsts*, 242–43. Also Herman A. Liebhafsky, *Silicones under the Monogram: A Story of Industrial Research* (New York: John Wiley & Sons, 1978), 67.

75   Lebhafsky, *Silicones under the Monogram*, 67–76.

76   *The Golden Nose*, a narrative history of the origins of silicone published and distributed by the Dow Corning Corporation. See also "The Silicones: A New Class of Synthetics Built on Sand," *Fortune*, May 1947, 104–111.

77   Warrick, *Forty Years of Firsts*, 242–43.

78   Ibid., 3–6, 9–14.

79   Ibid., 4–6.

80   Ibid., 21.

81   Ibid., 87–89, 194–98.

82   Ibid., 192–93. H. A. Liebhafsky, *Silicones under the Monogram*, 224–26 Rickover also visited General Electric in

Schenectady, New York, where a silicone polymer laboratory was active, but GE could not establish resin production quickly enough for military needs. GE later expanded production in Waterford, New York. On April 3, 1942, the Department of Commerce withdrew all patent applications for silicone products until the war ended. Security was more important than patent precedence.

83   Warrick, *Forty Years of Firsts*, 7–9.

84   Eldon E. Frisch, a Dow Corning consultant, called my attention to a brief letter appearing in *The British Medical Journal* on February 10, 1951, in which G. H. Darling and J. G. O. Spencer recall giving up paraffin as a syringe lubricant and adopting the newer and more functional silicone liquid.

85   Michael A. Bernstein, in *A Perilous Progress: Economists and Public Purpose in the Twentieth Century* (Princeton, NJ: Princeton University Press, 2001) 89–92.

86   Warrick, *Forty Years of Firsts*, 27–28. Author informed that although Earl Warrick claims to be the inventor of Silly Putty, James Wright of General Electric makes the same claim. Crayola LLC, current manufacturer and distributor of the product, uses Wright's story as the correct one.

87   Ibid., 88–94.

88   SightSavers, a trademark, are still marketed today. See Warrick, *Forty Years of Firsts,* for other postwar commercial products.

89   V. K. Rowe, H. C. Spencer, S. L. Bass, "Toxicological Studies on Certain Commercial Silicones," *Journal of Industrial Hygiene and Toxicology,* 30 (1948): 337–52.

90   Warrick, *Forty Years of Firsts,* 106.

Chapter 3

91   FDA Annual Report, 1933. Campbell served as FDA commissioner from 1924 to 1944.

92   Veronica D. DiConti, "The Federal Trade Commission," in George T. Kurian, *A Historical Guide to the U. S. Government,* (Oxford: Oxford University Press, 1998), 241–46.

93   "United States in "United States vs. Coca Cola Company," *US Reporter* 241 (October 1916): 279–280.

94   "United States vs. Coca Cola Company, *US Reporter* 241 (October 1916): 279–80.

95   Ibid., 265–90.

96   Young, "Three Southern Food and Drug Cases," 14–19.

97   John P. Swann, "Food and Drug Administration," Kurian, *A Historical Guide to the U. S. Government*, 248–54.

98   Biography.com: Harvey Washington Wiley died at his home in Washington, DC, on June 30, 1930, at the age of 86. He is buried in Arlington National Cemetery.

99   The campaign song story is related by Paul Johnson, *A History of the American People* (New York: HarperCollins, 1997), 751. Refer to Alan Brinkley, *The End of Reform: New Deal Liberalism in Recession and War* (New York: Alfred A. Knopf, 1995) for a discussion of Roosevelt's "swift and staccato action." Charles O. Jackson's *Food and Drug Legislation in the New Deal* (Princeton, NJ: Princeton University Press, 1970) offers account of the passage of the 1938 food law.

100   Jackson, *Food and Drug Legislation in the New Deal*, 3–8, 24–26.

101   Ibid., 9–15, 60–63.

102   James Harvey Young, "Sulfanilamide and Diethylene Glycol," in John Parascandola and James Whorton, *Chemistry and Modern Society: Historical Essays in Honor of Aaron J. Ihde* (Washington: American Chemical Society, 1983), 105–125. Harry Dowling, *Magic in a Bottle* (New York: Appleton-Century, 1943). Leonard Colebrook, *Lancet* 1 (1936): 1279–86. Perrin H. Long, *Journal of the American Medical Association* 108 (1937): 32–37. *New York Times*, December 17, 1936.

103   Editorial, *Journal of the American Medical Association*, 109 (1937): 1367.

104   His denial failed to prevent litigation and payment of significant fines.

105   Surveys to determine patient compliance with the filling of prescriptions or the fulfillment of a course of recommended

medication vary widely according to socioeconomic level and other factors, but they are rarely higher than 55%–65% and have been reported as low as 15%–20%.

106 Jackson, *Food and Drug Legislation in the New Deal*, 191.

107 Refer to Peter Hutt's writings for additional interpretation of significance of the 1938 Act.

108 Pliny, *Natural History*, vol. I-X, cited by Hutt, "A History of Government Regulation," N. F. Estrin and James M. Akerson, *Cosmetic Regulation in a Competitive Environment* (New York: Marcel Dekker, 2000), 1–2. Refer to Mr. Hutt's detailed history of the regulation of cosmetics, a topic beyond the scope of this work.

109 Jackson, *Food and Drug Regulation in the New Deal*, 145–49, 171–74, for derivation of the Wheeler-Lea Act and the scope of FTC jurisdiction over food and drugs.

110 Mark Pendergrast, *For God, Country, and Coca-Cola*, 191.

111 At war's end, the FDA and other regulatory agencies were handed another source of power in the form the Administrative Procedure Act (APA) 1946, legislation enacted for the purpose of improving government efficiency, likely encouraged by the recent extraordinary demonstration of efficient government while providing both materiel and manpower for winning a world war. In the words of one of its sponsors, U. S. Senator Pat McCarran, APA stood as a "bill of rights for the hundreds of thousands of Americans whose affairs are controlled or regulated by federal government agencies." The bill provided those agencies with the right to initiate regulations without prior legislative mandate.

Chapter 4

112 Author grateful for recollections of Allyn McDowell and Peter Randall, former residents of Dr. Brown. Frank McDowell, "James Barrett Brown, Obituary." *Plastic and Reconstructive Surgery* 48 (1971): 101–4.

113 Ibid., 103–4.

114 Silas A. Braley, "The Use of Silicones in Plastic Surgery, A Retrospective View." *Plastic and Reconstructive Surgery* 51 (1973).

115 Frank H. Lahey commented on the comparative use of Vitalium and silicone in a discussion of results using vitallium tubes in biliary surgery, *Annals of Surgery*, 124 (1946) 1020. R. Robert DeNicola, "Permanent Artificial (Silicone) Urethra," *Journal of Urology*, 63 (1950): 168–72.

116 Robert J. Prentiss, et al., "Testicular Prosthesis: Materials, Methods, and Results," *Journal of Urology*, 90 (1963): 208–9.

117 Ibid., 185. Also Braley, "The Use of Silicones in Plastic Surgery." Howard La Fay, "A Father's Last-Chance Invention Saves His Son," *Town Journal*, November 1956, 29–32.

118 See Warrick's *Forty Years of Firsts* for an extensive accounting of the activities of the Center for Aid to Medical Research.

119 Warrick, *Forty Years of Firsts*, 165–86.

120 Nancy Etcoff, *Survival of the Prettiest: The Science of Beauty*, (New York: Anchor Books, 2000), 2–5, 16–18, 30.

121 Mario Gonzalez-Ulloa, *The Creation of Aesthetic Plastic Surgery* (New York: Springer-Verlag, 1976).

122 John M. Goin and Marcia Kraft Goin, *Changing the Body: Psychological Effects of Plastic Surgery* (Baltimore: Williams & Wilkins, 1981). Robert M. Goldwyn, *The Patient and the Plastic Surgeon* (Boston: Little Brown & Co., 1991).

123 E. Berscheid and E. Walster, "Physical Attractiveness," *Advances in Experimental Social Psychology* 7 (1974). E. Berscheid and Steve Gangestad, "The Social Psychological Implications of Facial Physical Attractiveness," *Clinics in Plastic Surgery* 9 (1982): 289–96.

124 Etcoff, *Survival of the Prettiest*, 140–50.

125 Marilyn Yalom, *A History of the Breast* (New York: Alfred Knopf, 1997). Etcoff, *Survival of the Prettiest*, 187–90.

126 See David Halberstam's *The Fifties* (New York: Villard Books, 1993) for the emergence of Hugh Hefner's "Playboy culture." Images of advertisements for bust cream are

reproduced in Harry Hayes, *An Anthology of Plastic Surgery* (Rockville, MD: Aspen, 1986), 173.

127 Robert M. Goldwyn, "Vincenz Czerny and the Beginnings of Breast Reconstruction," *Plastic and Reconstructive Surgery* 61 (1978): 673–81.

128 J. P. Lalardrie and R. Mouly, "History of Mammaplasty," in Gonzalez-Ulloa, *The Creation of Aesthetic Plastic Surgery*, 135–44. Reuven K. Snyderman, "Reconstruction of the Breast After Surgery for Malignancy," in Robert M. Goldwyn, *Plastic and Reconstructive Surgery of the Breast* (Boston: Little Brown & Co., 1976): 465–84.

129 Ivalon is a derivative of polyvinyl alcohol. Polistan is a derivative of polyethylene, Etheron is a polyurethane, and Hydron is a derivative of polyglycomethacrylate.

130 Based on recollections of plastic surgeons who practiced at the time, among them Milton T. Edgerton, whom the author served as a resident-in-training at a time when patients were returning to exchange their porous sponge implants for a silicone device.

131 Based on personal recollections of former residents and partners, among them Roger Greenberg and Thomas Biggs.

132 Letter from Thomas D. Cronin to Silas Braley, January 12, 1961.

133 Letter from Ethel Mullison to Thomas Cronin, January 26, 1961. Dow Corning in 1961 was not a large enough company to maintain its own industrial hygiene and toxicology departments as it does today.

134 Correspondence between Frank Gerow or Thomas Cronin and Dow Corning engineers throughout 1961 and 1962 shown to the author while visiting Dow Corning.

135 Timmie Jean Lindsey recalled her experience for reporter Mimi Swartz in "The rise and fall of the implant—or how Houston went from an oil based economy to a breast based economy," *Texas Monthly Magazine*, August 1995.

136 Based on the recollections of Linda Alexander, wife of San Diego plastic surgeon John Alexander, who trained with Dr. Cronin.

137   Letter from Thomas D. Cronin to Silas Braley, April 15, 1962.

138   Dr. Thomas Biggs, who attended the congress, recalled the excitement in that room.

Chapter 5

139   Former New York Governor Hugh Carey recalled for the author the political career of his friend and colleague, James Delaney. A complete historiography of the McCarthy Era includes documentation from classified intercepts (see Venona Project) confirming that some of the senator's accused were in fact practicing communists but not necessarily practicing spies. Chemophobic theory prevails despite declining cancer death rates (see National Center for Health Statistics).

140   House Select Committee to Investigate the Use of Chemicals in Food Products, 81: H1310-6; 82: H 1362-1-A, SUDOC: Y4.F73/2: C42 & SUDOC Y4.F73/2: C42/2/pt. 1.

141   Based on data from the National Center for Health Statistics and from Population Reference Bureau Inc. as cited by William M. London and John W. Morgan, "Living Long Enough to Die of Cancer," *Priorities* (a publication of the American Council on Science & Health) 7 (1995) 6–9. Also refer to US Census Bureau, *Statistical Abstract of the United States,* 2003, Table HS-13, "Live Births, Deaths, Infant Deaths, and Maternal Deaths, 1900–2001, available at http://www.census.gov. Adam J. Lieberman, "Love Canal, 1978" in *Facts versus Fears,* Publication of the American Council on Science and Health, 1997, 14–15.

142   *Cancer Facts and Figures 2004,* American Cancer Society, New York, 2004. *Is There a Cancer Epidemic in the United States,* Publication of the American Council on Science and Health, 1995. During the twentieth century, certain cancers such as those developing in the stomach have diminished in frequency while others such as pancreatic cancer have increased.

143   Daniel Q. Haney, "Leukemia Mystery in the Desert," *San Diego Union-Tribune*, December 14, 2003. D. T. Max, "The Case of the Cherry Hill Cluster," *New York Times Magazine*, March 28, 2004.

144   Roper Center for Public Opinion Research, University of Connecticut.

145   U. S. House Committee, *Chemicals in Food Products*, 81: H1310-6, and 82: H1362-1-A (SUDOC: Y4.F73/2:C42/2/pt. 1. Maurice Natenberg, *The Legacy of Doctor Wiley and the Administration of his Food and Drug Act* (Chicago: Regent House, 1957), 109–137.

146   Natenberg, *The Legacy of Doctor Wiley*, 123–24. Hutt, *Regulation of Food Additives in the United States*, 7–8.

147   Natenberg, *The Legacy of Doctor Wiley*, 116.

148   H. M. Pachter, *Magic into Science: The Story of Paracelsus* (New York: Henry Schuman, 1951).

149   Hutt, *Regulation of Food Additives in the United States*, 7–8.

150   National Academy of Sciences, "The Use of Chemical Additives in Food Processing," NAS Publ. 398 (1956); 68 Stat. 511 (1954); 72 Stat. 1784 (1958); 74 Stat. 397 (1960).

151   The National Cancer Institute began conducting surveys of cancer incidence in 1937, leading ultimately to its SEER Program. This program combines data from all known cancer registries.

152   Peter Hutt, "Enactment of the 1958 Delaney Clause," *Food and Drug Law: Cases and Materials*, (Westbury, NY: The Foundation Press, 1991), 868–72.

153   J. Lynne Dodson, *"A Century of Oncology"* (Greenwich, CT: Greenwich Press, 1997), 50–53. M. F. W. Festing and E. M. C. Fisher, "Mighty Mice," *Nature* 404 (2000): 815. Brendan A. Maher, "Test Tubes With Tails," *The Scientist* 16 (2002): 22–24. Jean Holstein, *The First Fifty Years at The Jackson Laboratory*, (Bar Harbor, ME: The Jackson Laboratory, 1979).

154   Virginia Postrel interview of Bruce Ames, "Of Mice and Men: Finding Cancer's Causes," *Reason*, December 1991, 18–21.

155   Walter Williams, "Enjoy That Turkey Dinner; Just Don't Eat 3.8 Tons of It!" *Detroit News and Free Press,* July 7, 1991.

156   "Holiday Dinner Menu," American Council on Science and Health (http://www.acsh.org).

157   Bruce N. Ames, Margie Profet, Lois Swirsky Gold, "Nature's Chemicals and Synthetic Chemicals: Comparative Toxicology," *Proceedings of the National Academy of Sciences,* 87 (1990): 7782–85. Bruce N. Ames, Lois Swirsky Gold, "Chemical Carcinogenesis: Too Many Rodent Carcinogens," *Proceedings of the National Academy of Sciences,* 87 (1990): 7772–76.

158   Postrel, "Of Mice and Men," 18. William R. Havender, "The Science and Politics of Cyclamate," *The Public Interest* 71 (1983): 17–31. Elizabeth M. Whelan & Frederick, J. Stare, *Panic in the Pantry: Facts and Fallacies About the Food You Buy* (Buffalo, NY: Prometheus, 1992), 127, 132–3, 145–7, 154.

159   "Outrage of the Month: We Need the Delaney Anti-Cancer Clause," *Public Citizen Health Letter,* 8 (1992): 11.

160   Kristine Napier, "Reworking the Delaney Clause," *Priorities* (A Publication of the American Council on Science and Health), Spring 1992, 42–44. Ms. Streep later admitted that her fight against Alar had been based on shaky science. See Jesse Green, "What, Meryl Worry?" *New York Times,* July 25, 2004. EPA website continues to offer a detailed discussion of potential hazards from exposure to daminozide.

161   B. S. Oppenheimer, E. T. Oppenheimer, Arthur Purdy Stout, "Sarcomas Induced in Rats by Implanting Cellophane," *Proceedings of the Society of Experimental Biology & Medicine* 67 (1948): 33–34. B. S. Oppenheimer et al, "Malignant Tumors Resulting from Imbedding Plastics in Rodents," *Science* 118 (1953): 305–6. B. S. Oppenheimer et al., "Further Studies of Polymers as Carcinogenic Agents in Animals," *Cancer Research* 15 (1955): 333–40. For interpretation of solid state carcinogenesis, see K. Gerhard Brand, "Diversity and Complexity of Carcinogenic Processes: Conceptual Inferences from Foreign-Body Tumorigenesis," *Journal of the National*

Cancer Institute 57 (1976): 973–76. Toxic torts: a euphemism for product liability litigation.

Chapter 6

162 William Hazlitt, *Lectures on the English Comic Writers*, (New York: Wiley and Putnam, 1845), 2.

163 Peter Barton Hutt, "A History of Government Regulation of Adulteration and Misbranding of Medical Devices," *Food, Drug, Cosmetic Law Journal* 44 (1989): 99–105.

164 Andrew Gage, "The Development of the Implantable Cardiac Pacemaker," in Lilli Sentz et al., *Medical History in Buffalo 1846–1996: Collected Essays*, (Buffalo, NY: History of Medicine Collection, State University of New York–Buffalo, 1996), 247–56.

165 Richard E. McFayden, "Thalidomide in America: A Brush with Tragedy" in *Clio Medica* 2 (1976): 79–93. Also Philip Hilts, *Protecting America's Health: The FDA, Business and One Hundred Years of Regulation*, (Chapel Hill, NC: University of North Carolina, 2004), 143–63. Plastic surgeon Joseph E. Murray received the Nobel Prize in Physiology or Medicine in 1990 for his landmark achievements in organ transplantation, having transferred the first identical twin kidney in 1954.

166 Frances O. Kelsey, "Thalidomide Update: Regulatory Aspects, *Teratology* 38 (1988): 221–26.

167 Helen B. Taussig, "The Thalidomide Syndrome," *Scientific American* 207 (1962): 30–42.

168 Hubert Humphrey, senator from Minnesota and member of the Government Operations Committee conducted hearings into the thalidomide episode: US Congress, Senate, Committee Government Operations, Interagency Coordination in Drug Research and Regulation, 87th Congr., 2nd Sess., 1962, 75–82, 604–36.

169 Morton Mintz, "Heroine of the FDA Keeps Bad Drug Off the Market," *Washington Post*, July 15, 1962, 1. Morton Mintz, *By Prescription Only*, (Boston: Beacon Press, 1967).

170   *Congr. Record,* 115: 23,149, Aug. 11, 1969.

171   Hutt, "History of Government Regulation Of Medical Devices," 107–9. "Excerpts and Summary of a National Conference on Medical Devices," *Journal of the American Medical Association* 210 (1969): 1745.

172   Mary F. Hawkins, *Unshielded: The Human Cost of the Dalkon Shield* (Toronto: University of Toronto Press, 1997). Nicole J. Grant, *The Selling of Contraception: The Dalkon Shield Case, Sexuality, and Women's Autonomy* (Columbus: Ohio State University Press, 1992). Susan Perry and Jim Dawson, *Nightmare: Women and the Dalkon Shield* (New York: Macmillan, 1985).

173   Based on interviews with Dr. Charles A. Edwards in La Jolla, CA, and Peter Barton Hutt in Washington, DC. See also Hilts, *Protecting America's Health,* for evaluation of the Edwards tenure as FDA commissioner. See also Dr. Edward's autobiographical *Tough Choices: My Extraordinary Journey at the Heart of American Politics and Medicine* (privately published, 2005).

174   Perry and Dawson, *Nightmare,* 150–52.

175   Ibid., 160–80.

176   Based on author's discussions with executives of Dow Corning Corporation.

177   The author is grateful to Thomas Fitzgerald's widow, Joan, for locating two former GE associates of her husband, chemist Hart Lichtenwalner and attorney John Young, both of them helpful in recalling strategic corporate decisions made by GE in the 1970s.

178   J. B. Lynch recalled for the author early meetings of the Plastic and General Surgery Device Advisory Panel and the last panel meeting he attended in November 1988.

179   In 1999, ASPRS simplified its name to American Society of Plastic Surgeons (ASPS). For historical accuracy, the largest trade organization of surgeons certified by the American Board of Plastic Surgery will be referred to as ASPRS through 1998 and ASPS thereafter.

Chapter 7

180   This frequently quoted Latin phrase, which translates "First, do no harm," is abstracted from a longer admonition written by Hippocrates in *Of the Epidemics,* Book I: "As to diseases, make a habit of two things—to help, or at least to do no harm." For context, see Francis Adams, *The Genuine Works of Hippocrates,* (Baltimore: Williams & Wilkins, 1939), 98–141.

181   J. B. S. Haldane cited by William M. London and John W. Morgan, "Living Long Enough to Die of Cancer," *Priorities,* 7 (1995): 6.

182   Peter L. Bernstein, *Against the Gods: The Remarkable Story of Risk* (New York: John Wiley & Sons, 1996), 1–10.

183   September 11 air casualties courtesy of Google (total mortality that day including towers and the Pentagon now approaches 3,000). "Not Good at Risk, *The Economist* March 15, 2008. NTSB data for motor vehicle deaths fatalities range between three hundred and six hundred deaths per weekend, depending on season and weather conditions.

184   Bernstein, *Against the Gods,* 1–10.

185   Thomas D. Cronin and Frank J. Gerow, "Augmentation Mammaplasty: A New 'Natural Feel' Prosthesis," *Excerpta Medica International Congress* 66 (1963): 41–49.

186   Thomas D. Cronin, "Silicone Breast Implant: Historical Development," Chapter 36 in *Biomaterials in Plastic Surgery,* 552–54.

187   Ibid., 554.

188   Thomas D. Cronin and Roger L. Greenberg, "Our Experience with the Silastic Gel Breast Prosthesis" in *Plastic and Reconstructive Surgery,* 46 (1970): 1–7. Dr. Greenberg recalled for me that as of 1968 no patient had asked for removal of her breast implants.

189   H. G. Arion, "Prosthesis Retromammaires," *C.R. Soc. Fr. Gynecol.* 35: 427–31, 1965.

190   Garry S. Brody, "Fact and Fiction about Breast Implant "Bleed," *Plastic and Reconstructive Surgery* 60 (1977): 615–16.

191   First reported in Scottsdale, Arizona, in November 1975. James L. Baker, "Augmentation Mammaplasty," in J. Q. Owsley and R. A. Peterson, *Symposium on Aesthetic Surgery of the Breast,* (St. Louis: C. V. Mosby, 1978), 256–63. A comparison study of this kind would not be approved by a human subjects institution review board today because of a concern that most patients would notice an asymmetric result and demand reoperation.

192   Current thinking about capsule contraction takes into account an invisible biofilm that surrounds every implanted device. Populated with bacteria from the body's own microflora, attorneys have long ignored this or any other issue they can't blame on a corporation.

193   Ross Rudolph, Joe Utley, and Marilyn Woodward, "Contractile Fibroblasts in a Painful Pacemaker Pocket," *Annals of Thoracic Surgery,* 31 (1981): 373–76. Ross Rudolph, Jerrold Abraham, Thomas Vecchione, Seven Guber, and Marilyn Woodward, "Myofibroblasts and Free Silicon Around Breast Implants," *Plastic and Reconstructive Surgery* 62 (1978): 185–96. M. G. Wickham, Ross Rudolph, Jerrold L. Abraham, "Silicon Identification in Prosthesis-Associated Fibrous Capsules," *Science* 199 (1978): 437–39. Robert Gayou and Ross Rudolph, "Capsular Contraction Around Silicone Mammary Prostheses," *Annals Plastic Surgery* 2 (1979): 62–71.

194   Boyd R. Burkhardt, "Comparing Contracture Rates: Probability Theory and the Unilateral Contracture," *Plastic and Reconstructive Surgery,* 74 (1984): 527–29. Because of his preference for saline-filled implants, Dr. Burkhardt would later be invited by the FDA to speak at one its hearings, even taken to dinner the night before by an FDA official. But his testimony included no specific criticism of gel implants. Don McGhan recalled for the author the origins of low-bleed elastomer shells. Rudolph's conclusions were counter to industry position despite Dow Corning and Inamed providing his funding.

195   D. G. Bower and C. B. Radlauer, "Breast Cancer after Pro-
      phylactic Subcutaneous Mastectomies and Reconstruction
      with Silastic Prosthesis," *Plastic Reconstructive Surgery* 44
      (1969): 541. W. J. Benavent, "Treatment of Bilateral Breast
      Carcinomas in a Patient with Silicone Gel Breast Implants:
      Case Report," *Plastic Reconstructive Surgery* 51 (1973): 588. W.
      Alvarez, "Operations on Bosoms Dangerous," *Los Angeles
      Times,* January 11, 1954. W. S. Kiskadden, "Operations on
      Bosoms Dangerous," *Plastic Reconstructive Surgery* 15 (1955):
      79. John E. Hoopes, Milton T. Edgerton, William Shelley,
      "Organic Synthetics and Augmentation Mammaplasty:
      Their Relation to Breast Cancer," Plastic Reconstructive
      Surgery 39 1967): 263–69.

196   June Marchant, "Breast Prostheses," *Lancet* 2 (1975): 187–88.

197   Nigel Paneth et al., "Origins and Early Development of the
      Case-Control Study: Part 1, Early Evolution," *Soz Praven-
      tivmed* 47 (2002): 282–88. Nigel Paneth et al., "Origins
      and Early Development of the Case-Control Study: Part 2,
      The Case-Control Study from Lane-Claypon to 1950," *Soz
      Praventivmed* 47 (2002): 359–65.

198   Richard Doll, "Cohort Studies: History of the Method, 1.
      Prospective Cohort Studies," *Soz Praeventivmed* 46 (2001):
      75–86. Richard Doll, Cohort Studies: History of the Meth-
      od, 2. Retrospective Cohort Studies," *Soz Praeventivmed* 46
      (2001): 152–60.

199   Drs. Brody and Deapen recalled for this author the plan-
      ning and design of their epidemiologic study.

200   D. M. Deapen, M. C. Pike, J. T. Casagrande, G. S. Brody,
      "The Relationship between Breast Cancer and Augmen-
      tation Mammaplasty: An Epidemiologic study," *Plastic
      Reconstructive Surgery* 77 (1986): 361.

201   Author examined evolution of PIDs published by Hey-
      er-Schulte between 1972 and 1984. Reporting for the *New
      York Times,* June 5, 2011, Gina Kolata cited studies showing
      an average seventy side effects listed for drugs, "linguis-
      tic toxicity" according to one observer. Even after the FDA

recommended guidelines for listing side effects, the average number increased from sixty-seven to ninety-four.

202   James L. Baker, Roger J. Bartels, William M. Douglas, "Closed Compression for Rupturing a Contracted Capsule Around a Breast Implant," *Plastic Reconstructive Surgery* 58 (1976): 137–41.

203   Thomas M. Biggs, Jean Cukier, L. Fabian Worthing, "Augmentation Mammaplasty: A Review of 18 Years," *Plastic Reconstructive Surgery* 69 (1982): 445–50.

204   Mrs. Lindsay spoke about her experience with breast implants at a time when ASPRS was asking satisfied patients to speak out. Mrs. Lindsay was also urged by lawyers to sue but always refused. See Mimi Swartz, *Texas Monthly Magazine,* August 1995. A contemporary Google search yields several fictitious interviews claiming she lived a life of misery because of breast implants.

Chapter 8

205   Policy explained to author and other plastic surgeons at a meeting in Santa Barbara, CA, in July 1989.

206   Warwick, *Forty Years of Firsts,* 288–90.

207   Ibid., 290–92.

208   Deborah Tedford, "Revelation Old News to East Texas Woman," *Houston Chronicle,* February 11, 1992. Joseph Nocera, "Fatal Litigation," *Fortune* 32 (1995): 60–78.

209   Ms. Barbara Canetti facilitated an email exchange between the author and Mr. Mithoff regarding *Corley vs. Dow Corning.*

210   "History of ASPRS," *Plastic and Reconstructive Surgery,* 94 (1994): 72A–73A.

211   Ibid., 74A. Also based on the author's interview of Dr. Rex Peterson. Dr. Peterson defied not only the FTC but also his own organization's attorneys, believing they were in conflict of interest because of their concurrent service to other professional organizations. Dr. Mark Gorney recalled for the author his viewing of the taped comments of Commissioner Michael Pertschuk.

212 William Porterfield, "Comments of the American Society of Plastic and Reconstructive Surgery on the Proposed Classification of Inflatable Breast Prosthesis (Docket 78N – 2653) and Silicone Gel-Filled Breast Prosthesis (Docket 78N – 2654)." By convention, the word "prosthesis" is applied to devices affixed to the body's surface and the word "implant" to devices imbedded within the body.

213 H. D. Kagan, "Sakurai Injectable Silicone Formula," *Archives of Otolaryngology* 78 (1962): 663.

214 Letter to Harry D. Dingman, Dow Corning, from Franklin D. Clark, Bureau of Regulatory Compliance, FDA, December 9, 1964. Investigational Drug Application: Dow Corning MDX 4-4011. Medical Fluid for Tissue Augmentation by Injection Except for Mammary Area: Dow Corning Form FD 1571, submitted June 8, 1965. The following investigators participated in the first liquid silicone protocol: Franklin L. Ashley, UCLA; Ralph Blocksma, Grand Rapids, Michigan; Reed O. Dingman, University of Michigan; Milton T. Edgerton, Johns Hopkins Hospital; Dicran Goulian Jr., New York-Cornell; Francis L. Lederer, University of Illinois; Joseph E. Murray, Harvard University; Norman Orentreich, Thomas D. Rees, New York University.

215 Dr. Balkin recalled his studies of liquid silicone for the author and also provided his forty-year follow-up clinical results. See also S. W. Balkin, "The Fluid Silicone Prosthesis," in *Symposium on Implants in Foot Surgery: Clinics in Podiatry* 1 (1984): 145–64. S. W. Balkin and L. Kaplan, "Injectable Silicone and the Diabetic Foot: A 25-Year Report," *The Foot* 1 (July 1991): 83–88.

216 Reports of silicone mastitis appeared in medical journals throughout the world. In Great Britain, the term "prosthetogenic mastitis" was coined. See W. S. C. Symmers, "Silicone Mastitis in Topless Waitresses," *British Medical Journal* 3 (1968): 19–22. Dr. Kopf recalled for the author his personal efforts securing restrictive legislation against injectable silicone. *Nevada Revised Statutes Annotated* 15 @ 202.248

(1975). California Business and Professions Code Div. 2, Ch. 5, Art. 12 @ 2251 (1976). Noteworthy is the FDA's review and approval of silicone fluid for ophthalmologic applications while at the same time attributing serious illnesses to silicone gel breast implants.

217   Letter from FDA Commissioner James L. Goddard to Harry D. Dingman, Dow Corning on October 18, 1967. Statement of Mel Nelson, Medical Products Manager, Dow Corning: "We have decided to suspend efforts to obtain approval because after several months of work, we have not been able to devise a workable system of controls that would preclude misuse of the product."

218   Amendment to IND 22702 Submitted by Dow Corning Corporation, September 2, 1977. Letter to A. H. Rathjen, Dow Corning Corporation from Joseph L. Hacket, Bureau of Medical Devices, FDA, January 18, 1979.

219   Dennis M. Deapen, Malcolm C. Pike, John T. Casagrande, Garry S. Brody, "The Relationship Between Breast Cancer and Augmentation Mammaplasty: An Epidemiologic Study," in *Plastic Reconstructive Surgery* 77 (1986): 361–67.

220   Lynn Rosenberg, Discussion of "The Relationship Between Breast Cancer and Augmentation Mammaplasty: An Epidemiologic Study," *Plastic Reconstructive Surgery* 77 (1986): 368.

221   According to Gene Jakubczak, Dow Corning provided twenty-five thousand dollars to the University of Southern California for continuation of the Deapen-Brody study.

222   Alison Frankel, "From Pioneers to Profits: The Splendid Past and the Muddled Present of Breast Implant Litigation," *The American Lawyer,* June 1992, 82–91. Joseph Nocera, "Fatal Litigation" Part I, *Fortune,* October 16, 1995, 60–64.

223   Ibid., 64–66. Dow Corning later explained that Heggers' proposal was not funded because reviewers believed sufficient evidence showed silicone to have little effect on immunity.

224   Frankel, "From Pioneers to Profits," *American Lawyer,* 84.

225 Sybil Norden Goldrich, "Restoration Drama: A Cautionary Tale by a Woman Who Had Breast Implants after Mastectomy," *Ms.* June 1988, 20–22. Sidney Wolfe's presentation on CNN in October 1988 was followed by numerous restatements of his warning. See also testimony before the FDA Advisory Panel for General and Plastic Devices, November 22, 1988.

226 Based on author's review of tapes and transcripts from the hearing. Also in October 2004, Dr. Lynch shared with the author his memories and impressions of the General and Plastic Surgery Device Advisory Panel meeting on November 22, 1988.

227 Frankel, "From Pioneers to Profits," 87.

228 Proceedings of the FDA Advisory Panel, November 22, 1988.

229 Robert Singer to Norman Hugo, "Report of the Implant Product Development Committee, ASAPS, March 1, 1982.

230 FDA Commissioner Frank Young to Sidney Wolfe, November 22, 1988. The letter is not copied to the FDAs Dr. Nirval Mishra, who might have benefited from the commissioner's interpretation.

231 Based on notes recorded following conversations between Robert Rylee and the author in July 1989.

Chapter 9

232 As told to Dr. Garry Brody by Sybil Goldrich of Command Trust Network.

233 Goldrich, "Restoration Drama," 20–21.

234 At the time there was one source of syringes advertised to be free of silicone . . . in Germany.

235 K. Miyoshi, T. Miyamura, Y. Kobayashi, T. Itakura, K. Nishijo, M. Higashibara, H. Shiragami, F. Ohno, "Hyper-gammaglobuilinemia by Prolonged Adjuvanticity in Man: Disorders Developed after Augmentation Mammaplasty," *Ijishimpo (Japan Medical Journal)* 2112 (1964): 9–14. Immunologists sometimes use adjuvants to strengthen

an immune response in rodents but not humans; an adjuvant can produce excessive immunity damaging to the host.

236 K. Yoshida, "Post Mammoplasty Disorder as an Adjuvant Disease of Man," *Shikoku Acta Med* 29/4 (1973): 318–32. Yasuo Kumagai, Abe Chiyuki, Yuchi Shiokawa, "Scleroderma After Cosmetic Surgery: Four Cases of Human Adjuvant Disease," *Arthritis and Rheumatism* 22 (1979): 532–37. Hirobumi Kondo, Yasuo Kumagai, Yuichi Shiokawa, "Scleroderma Following Cosmetic Surgery ("Adjuvant Disease"): A Review of Nine Cases Reported in Japan," in *Current Topics in Rheumatology: Systemic Sclerosis (Scleroderma)* (New York: Gower Publ. Ltd., 1981), 135–37.

237 The author pursued this question at the time of the controversy. Patients with silicone mastitis and associated wound problems were sometimes seen at UC–San Diego Medical Center. None reported rheumatic symptoms. Regular communication with Dr. Kopf in Las Vegas confirmed the same finding. Never published, our combined inquiries involved an estimated twenty to thirty patients.

238 Barry F. Uretsky, James O'Brien, Eugene H. Courtiss, Martin D. Becker, "Augmentation Mammaplasty Associated with a Severe Systemic Illness," *Annals of Plastic Surgery* 3 (1979): 445–47. Sheryl A. van Nunen, Paul A. Gatenby, and Antony Basten, "Post-Mammoplasty Connective Tissue Disease," *Arthritis and Rheumatism* 25 (1982): 694–97 (The author was asked by editor Nathan Zvaifler to review the van Nunen manuscript before publication).

239 Steven R. Weiner and Harold E. Paulus, "Chronic Arthropathy Occurring after Augmentation Mammaplasty," *Plastic Reconstructive Surgery* 77 (1986): 185–87.

240 Michael H. Weisman, MD, Thomas R. Vecchione, Daniel Albert, Lawrence T. Moore, Mary Rose Mueller, "Connective-Tissue Disease Following Breast Augmentation: A Preliminary Test of the Human Adjuvant Disease Hypothesis," *Plastic Reconstructive Surgery* 82 (1986): 626–30.

241 Newsletters issued by the Command Trust Network featured only physicians and scientists who supported links between silicone and disease, Dr. Weiner among them. They disparaged any source doubting complications from silicone exposure. In their view, silicone gel was nothing less than one of the most toxic materials known to mankind.

242 Alicia Ault, "Health-Care Watchdog," *Health Watch* July/August 1991, 47–51. Dennis L. Breo, "Sidney Wolfe, MD—Healing the System or Just Raising Hell?" *Journal of the American Medical Association* 266 (1991): 1131–33.

243 Milton Copulos, "It's Effective—But is it Safe?" *Reason,* March 1985, 24–32.

244 Sybil Goldrich, "A Special Memo from Command Trust Network," September 24, 1993.

245 Ms. Finestone recalled her experiences for the author in 2004.

246 "Warning Letter" sent by certified mail by Ronald Johnson, director, Office of Compliance and Surveillance, Center for Devices and Radiologic Health, FDA to Dr. Alan Broughton, Antibody Assay Laboratories, Santa Ana, CA, August 19, 1992.

247 Kimber White, Sanders, V. M, Barnes, D. W., Shopp, G. M., Munson, A. E., Imunotoxicological Investigations in the Mouse: General Approach and Methods, *Drug and Chemical Toxicology* 8 (1985): 299–322.

248 See http://www.fumento.com for Michael Fumento, "Implant Tests Cashing in on Junk Science, February 27, 1996.

249 Neil L. Rosenberg, "The Neuromythology of Silicone Breast Implants," *Neurology* 46 (1996) 308–314. See http://www.humanticsfoundation.com for Bernard M. Patten, *Memoir of a Junk Scientist,* in which the author defends but reveals the scientific weakness of his neurologic disease thesis.

250 Based on data maintained by the American Board of Plastic Surgery and the American Society of Plastic Surgery.

251 Members of the Silicone Implant Research Committee met with Dr. Cole in January 1990 at ASPRS offices in Arlington Heights, IL.

Chapter 10

252   Taken from Mr. Hilts' comments at a meeting of The Food and Drug Law Institute in 1994.

253   Based on a transcript of the December 10, 1990, broadcast of *Face to Face with Connie Chung*. Available on www.yukonmom47.tripod.com, website of the Implant Veterans of Toxic Exposure.

254   Ms. Chung's opinion of her broadcast preceded a rebroadcast of the December 2, 1990, exposé on November 8, 1991, timed by CBS to appear just four days before the FDA began its hearing on breast implant safety data.

255   "First National Survey Asks Women How They Feel About Breast Implants," released by ASPRS, November 1990, based on results of survey conducted by Market Facts, Chicago, IL.

256   Transcript of *Sally Jesse Raphael Show*, January 15, 1991.

257   Giovanna Breu, "My Breast Implant Disaster," *People*, March 2, 1982, 56–60.

258   Bonnie Winters, "One Woman's Case History of a Nightmare," *Kentucky Post*, July 26, 1990. Nancy Benec, "FDA Accused of Downplaying Possible Breast-Implant Risk," as reported by the Associated Press in the *Orange County Register*, April 28, 1991. Sandra Blakeslee, "Carcinogen Found in Milk of Mom Who Has Implants," *New York Times*, June 2, 1991.

259   ASPRS was told by its consultants that Fenton had placed more than two thousand stories in newspapers throughout the nation within a few weeks, mostly based on false science.

260   Recalled by Garry S. Brody, MD, following a conversation with Sybil Goldrich.

261   Susan D. Moeller, *Compassion Fatigue: How the Media Sell Disease, Famine, War, and Death*, (New York City: Routledge, 1999).

262   Jack Raso, "Nutrition-Related 'Credentialing' Organizations: The Good, the Bad, and the Abysmal, *Priorities 7*

(1999): 31–34. William H. London, "60 Minutes on Health: Picks and Pans," http://www.acsh.org, January 1, 2000.

263 Yes, the Flat Earth Society endures. See http://flatearthsociety.org for articles such as "Even Pictures from Space Show Only Mild Curvature" by Malcolm Ritter, "e=mcWhat?: Americans Still Don't Know Much About Science," Associated Press as reported in *San Diego Union-Tribune,* July 3, 2002, F1, F4.

264 June Kronholz, "Economic Time Bomb: U. S. Teens Are Among Worst in Math," *Wall Street Journal,* December 7, 2004, B1–B3. Diane Ravitch, "Failing the Wrong Grades," *New York Times,* March 15, 2005.

265 "High Tech Brain Drain," *Wall Street Journal Review & Outlook,* May 5, 2005, based on data from the Higher Education Research Institute at UCLA.

266 Kathy McNamara-Meis, "It Seemed We Had It All Wrong," *Forbes Media Critic,* Winter 1996, 40–49.

267 Virginia I. Postrel, "Policy Bust," *Reason* March 1992, 4–6.

268 John Stossel, *Give Me a Break,* New York (Harper Collins, 2004), 104–7.

269 Ms. Kolata was interviewed by the author in March 2005.

270 Gina Kolata and Barry Meier, "Implant Lawsuits Create A Medical Rush to Cash In," *New York Times,* September 18, 1995. Mark Dowie, "What's Wrong With the New York Times Science Reporting?" *Nation,* July 6, 1998.

271 Kathy McNamara-Meis, "It Seemed We Had it All Wrong," *Forbes Media Critic,* Winter, 1996, 45. Frank Vasey and Josh Feldstein, *The Silicone Breast Implant Controversy: What Women Need to Know,* 1993, in which the following symptoms all associated with a "silicone disease" are listed: "suicidal depression, mental lapses, pain in gall bladder, loss of sex drive, chronic exhaustion, night sweats, insomnia, flu-like symptoms, mouth ulcers, poor concentration, memory failure, abdominal pain, pain in the groin, fluid retention, asthma-like wheezing, frequent urination, unexplained rashes, arthritis, difficulty

swallowing, swollen lymph glands, dry eyes/mouth, short-
ness of breath, difficulty breathing, crushing chest pain,
muscle weakness, gallbladder pain, gallbladder polyps,
scleroderma, rheumatic disease, human adjuvant disease, auto-immune disease, connective tissue disease,
emotional breakdown, appetite loss, heart attack symptoms, depression, hypertension, tremors, weight loss,
weight gain, joint pain, dizzy spells, hair loss, numbness
in limbs and head, burning, tingling, hardness of the
breasts, gastrointestinal problems, urinary tract problems, irritable bowel, sleep disturbances, redness of the
palms (palmar erythema), blurred vision, neck pain, fibro-
myalgia, rheumatoid arthritis, low-grade fevers, nausea,
tender points on body, kidney failure, facial pain, double
vision, vertigo, pleurisy, lung pain, migraine headaches,
cold sensitivity, multiple sclerosis, small areas of muscle
that quiver, twitches, back pain, neck pain [again], chronic
cough, multiple environmental allergies, chronic bron-
chitis, lupus, Sjogren's syndrome, heart palpitations, joint
inflammation, clumsiness, and morning stiffness." As
cited in Bernstein, "The Breast Implant Fiasco," 481. The
story of a diagnosis made from behind a desk was told by
a woman who didn't even have breast implants but sought
Dr. Vasey's opinion (it was "silicone disease") and asks to
remain anonymous.

Chapter 11

272 Peter Hutt quoted by *New York Times* journalist Peter J.
     Hilts in "New Chief Vows New Vitality at FDA," *New York
     Times*, February 27, 1991.

273 Randi Henderson, "Meet David Kessler," *Hopkins Medical
     News*, Winter 1993, 61–68.

274 Peter Brimelow and Leslie Spencer, "Just Call Me 'Doc,' "
     Forbes, November 22, 1993, 108. Maggie Mahar, "Under
     a Microscope, FDA Chief David Kessler Keeps His Cool,"
     Barrons, March 2, 1992.

275   Henderson, "Meet David Kessler," 66–67. Herbert Burkholz, "A Shot in the Arm for the FDA," *New York Times Magazine,* June 30, 1991, 15–16.

276   "Running the code" is a resident physician's euphemism for directing life resuscitation following cardiac arrest.

277   Henderson, "Meet David Kessler," 64.

278   Brimelow and Spencer, "Just Call Me 'Doc," *Forbes,* November 22, 1993, 108–110.

279   Among observers who likened David Kessler to Harvey Wiley was journalist Philip Hilts, who had long covered the FDA for the *New York Times.* See Philip J. Hilts, *Protecting America's Health: The FDA, Business, and One Hundred Years of Regulation,* (New York: Alfred Knopf, 2003), 257–61. David Kessler reflects on the circumstances of his nomination and appointment. See David A. Kessler, *A Question of Intent: A Great American Battle with a Deadly Industry,* (New York: Public Affairs, 2001), 1–9.

280   Hilts, *Protecting America's Health,* 257–58. David A. Kessler, *A Question of Intent,* 5–8.

281   Herbert Burkholz, "A Shot in the Arm for the FDA," *New York Times,* June 30, 1991, 15. All other press quotes cited by Henderson in "Meet David Kessler," 63.

282   Henderson, "Meet David Kessler," 63–64.

283   Hilts, *Protecting America's Health,* 255.

284   Ibid., 256.

285   Kessler, *A Question of Intent,* 11–15.

286   Hilts, *Protecting America's Health,* 261–62.

287   Kessler, *A Question of Intent,* 21–25. The nation's bakers, through the American Bakers Association, has long quarreled with the FDA about use of the terms "fresh bread" and "fresh-baked bread," the established rule being that "fresh-baked" is permissible but "fresh" is not because of preservatives present in commercially sold bread, specifically calcium propionate which inhibits the growth of mold. (Reported by Cindy Skrzycki, "FDAs Fresh Stand on Rule Baffles Bakers," *Washington Post,* Oct. 15, 2002).

288   David Grogan and Marilyn Balamaci, "Food Fight: Doctor, Lawyer, FDA Chief," *People,* June 24, 1991, 82–83.

289   Kessler, *A Question of Intent,* 19.

290   Based on interviews with former FDA Commissioner Charles Edwards in La Jolla, CA, and former FDA General Counsel Peter Barton Hutt in Washington, DC. See also Dr. Kessler's *A Question of Intent* in which he is as forthright about criticism as Dr. Wiley was in his own autobiography.

291   "Conference on Silicone in Medical Devices," February 1–2, 1991, in Baltimore, MD, program announcement of the Center for Devices and Radiologic Health, FDA, US DHHS.

292   Nirmal K. Mishra DVM, "Hypothesis for a Potential Mechanism of Silicone-Induced Carcinogenesis," *Conference Proceedings: Silicone in Medical Devices,* (Center for Devices and Radiologic Health: FDA, December 1991), 155–68. Dennis M. Deapen, DPH, "Breast Cancer and Augmentation Mammaplasty," *Conference Proceedings: Silicone in Medical Devices,* (Center for Devices and Radiologic Health: FDA, December 1991), 169–74.

293   Panel Discussion, *Conference Proceedings: Silicone in Medical Devices,* (Center for Devices and Radiologic Health: FDA, December 1991), 273–300.

294   Frank L. Ashley, "A New Type of Breast Prosthesis: Preliminary Report," *Plastic Reconstructive Surgery* 45 (1970): 45. For clinical results, refer to Vincent R. Pennisi, "Long-Term Use of Polyurethane Breast Prostheses: A 14-Year Experience," *Plastic Reconstructive Surgery* 86 (1990): 368–71, and T. Roderick Hester et al., "A Five-year Experience with Polyurethane-Covered Mammary Prostheses for Treatment of Capsular Contracture, Primary Augmentation Mammoplasty, and Breast Reconstruction," *Clinics in Plastic Surgery* 15 (1988): 569–85. Carolyn L. Kerrigan, "Report on the Meme Breast Implant: Prepared for the Minister of Health and Welfare Canada," May 1989.

295   "Breast implants linked to risk of liver cancer: 750,000 women use suspect devices," *San Francisco Examiner,* April

14, 1991. Richard H. Cardy, "Carcinogenicity and Chronic Toxicity of 2,4-Toluenediamine in Fischer 344 Rats," *Journal of the National Cancer Institute* 62 (1979): 1107–16.

296 Letter to members from ASPRS President H. Bruce Williams citing meeting with Robert L. Sheridan, April 19, 1991. Letter to Garry S. Brody from Elizabeth D. Jacobson, April 24, 1991 (and issued as a press release on April 25, 1991).

297 Alison Frankel, "From Pioneers to Profits," *The American Lawyer,* June 1992, 88–89.

298 Transcript of General and Plastic Surgery Advisory Panel proceedings June 31, 1991, provided by Olga Papach Transcription Services. Garry L. Carter, VP and General Manager for Plastic Surgery, Surgitek, announced on July 9, 1991, that because the FDA had asked on June 28 for more testing, their filing of a Pre-Market Approval Application (PMAA) would be postponed pending completion of those tests. This would effectively remove the product from the market because without a PMAA filed by David Kessler's deadline, July 9, 1991, no manufacturer could lawfully continue to market implants.

299 July 8, 1991, press release announcing shipment of two PMAAs to FDA from Dow Corning Corporation.

300 Sandra Blakeslee, "Unapproved Breast Implant Seized," *New York Times,* July 31, 1991.

301 "History of ASPRS, *Plastic and Reconstructive Surgery,* September 1994, 93A. Also based on the author's conversations with Norman Cole.

302 Letter from Robert L. Sheridan, director of the Office of Device Evaluation, to Bailey Lipscomb, director of Clinical and Regulatory Affairs, Dow Corning, September 13, 1991.

303 ASPRS staffer Zan Lofgren recalled that Jon Kent of Kent & O'Connor organized additional Washington consultants, who included Stuart Pape and Mark Heller of Patton, Boggs, and Blow (Democratic); Roger Stone of Black, Manafort, Stone, & Kelly (Republican); Bobbie Lawrie served as

in-house crisis manager/PR consultant; and Porter Novelli served as outside PR consultant.

304 Patients were advised to say they paid for their own travel, but ASPRS later decided to reimburse patients but not doctors, accruing expenses totaling $248,000, a fact not overlooked by the press.

305 Alison Frankel, "From Pioneers to Profits," *The American Lawyer,* June 1992, 87–89.

306 As reported in *Breast Implant Bulletin,* November 11, 1991, 1 (a newsletter published by ASPRS).

307 Proceedings of General and Plastic Surgery Devices Advisory Panel, November 12, 1991, 2–5.

308 Events of this hearing based on notes taken by the author at the time. Some time later, a letter from Melvin Sabshin, MD, to David A. Kessler, MD, on March 3, 1993, made clear the position of 38,000 members of the American Psychiatric Association—"We already know that most women who receive implants are satisfied with the result"—and cautioned the FDA against conducting a rumored study protocol that would restrict half the enrolled subjects from receiving an implant.

309 Proceedings of the General and Plastic Surgery Device Advisory Panel, November 12, 1991, 9–26, 239–299, 323–324, 372–374.

310 Proceedings of the General and Plastic Surgery Devices Advisory Panel, November 13, 1991, 416–19.

311 Ibid., November 13, 220–31.

312 Ibid., November 14, 371–77. The terms "prosthesis" and "implant" are often used interchangeable, but by convention, implants are imbedded, prostheses are worn at the body surface.

313 Ibid., November 14, 272–74, 275–77. When the author interviewed Dr. Krizek in May 2005, he pointed out that his Silastic wrist implant remains functional and intact after long use.

314 Bernstein, "The Breast Implant Fiasco," 473–76. Marcia

Angell, *Science on Trial* (New York: W. W. Norton, 1966), 55–56, 118–25.

315   Bernstein, "The Breast Implant Fiasco," 472–74. Letter from Norman Anderson to David Kessler, December 12, 1991.

316   Dan M. Hayes to David A. Kessler, December 27, 1991.

317   Former DHHS Secretary Louis Sullivan recalled for the author his role in the breast implant moratorium decision for the author during a May 2005 interview.

Chapter 12

318   Dr. Kessler's often-used tire analogy appeared in print in the *New England Journal of Medicine* on June 18, 1992.

319   Statement of Congresswoman Marilyn Lloyd before the General and Plastic Surgery Device Advisory Panel, November 13, 1991.

320   David A. Kessler, "Statement on Silicone Gel Breast Implants" January 6, 1992. Accompanying press statement by Susan Cruzan appeared in *HHS News*, US Department of Health and Human Services, January 6, 1992.

321   See http://www.kirstytv.com, "Breast Implants Gone Wrong, Sybil Goldrich Warns Women." Marilyn Elias, "MDs still may be offering gel breast implants," *USA Today*, January 14, 1992. Letter from ASPRS President Norman Cole to FDA Commissioner David Kessler, January 15, 1992.

322   A spreading inkblot depicting dispersal of silicone gel throughout the body appeared on NBC network broadcasts in 1992. Transcript of Diane Rehm's interview of David Kessler January 8, 1992, from Diversified Reporting Services Inc., 918 16th St., N.W. Ste 803, Washington, DC 20006.

323   "Wise Time Out on Breast Implants," Editorial, *New York Times*, January 8, 1992, A14. "Science Abdicates," *Wall Street Journal*, January 9, 1992. Peter Huber, "A Woman's Right to Choose," *Forbes*, February 17, 1992. "WLF Blasts FDA Bias," *Washington Legal Foundation News*, January 20, 1991.

324   Surveys conducted periodically by ASPRS.

325   Norman Cole to David Kessler, April 17, 1992. David Kessler to Norman Cole, April 21, 1992.

326   John A. Byrne, *Informed Consent* (New York: McGraw Hill, 1996), 181–85. Joseph Nocera, "Fatal Litigation" in *Fortune,* October 16,1995.

327   Numerous conversations occurred between the author and Ralph Cook on epidemiologic investigations pertinent to silicone issues.

328   D. M. Gott and J. J. B. Tinkler, "Evaluation of Evidence for an Association between the Implantation of Silicones and Connective Tissue Disease," Medical Device Directorate, December 1994. The author also draws from notes taken during a 1994 meeting with Susanna M. Ludgate, MD, Medical Device Directorate, Department of Health, London, UK.

329   Author could not confirm rumors that Commissioner Kessler had been ordered to attend. Dr. E. James Potchen, University Distinguished Professor and chairman, Department of Radiology, Michigan State University.

330   Statement of Tennessee Representative Marilyn Lloyd before the FDA General and Plastic Surgery Devices Panel, February 19, 1992.

331   Dr. Zvaifler, a UCSD colleague, recalled for the author Dr. Sergent's hearing testimony.

332   Russell Seitz, "Congressional Math," *Wall Street Journal,* November 11, 2005, in which he calls attention to the fact that the very few scientists in Congress, only eight at the time of his tabulation, are always outnumbered by the attorneys.

333   David A. Kessler, "The Basis for the FDA's Decision on Breast Implants," *New England Journal of Medicine* 326 (1992): 1713–15. Marcia Angell, "Breast Implants—Protection or Paternalism," *New England Journal of Medicine* 326 (1992): 1695–96. Hans Berkel, Dale C. Birdsell, Heather Jenkins, "Breast Augmentation: A Risk Factor For Breast Cancer?" *New England Journal of Medicine* 326 (1992): 1649–53.

334 John A. Byrne, *Informed Consent*, (New York: McGraw-Hill, 1996), 175.

335 Herbert B. Newberg, *Newberg on Class Actions* (New York: McGraw-Hill, 1992), I-22, I-23.

336 Joseph Nocera, "Fatal Litigation," *Fortune*, October 16, 1995, 74–80. Alison Frankel, "From Pioneers to Profits," *The American Lawyer*, June 1992, 82–90.

337 In 2013, the Kentucky Supreme Court voted unanimously to disbar Chesley for "knowingly participating in a scheme to skim millions in excess attorney's fees from unknowing clients." *Wall Street Journal*, "Justice for the Disaster Master," August 12, 2014.

338 Christopher Palmeri, "A Texas Gunslinger," *Forbes*, July 3, 1995, 42–45. Dr. Melvin Spira provided the anecdote about Dr. Cronin politely receiving subpoenas by the hundreds.

339 *Johnson v. Bristol-Myers Squibb Co.* (91-021770) (Texas Harris County District Court), December 18, 1992 cited by David E. Bernstein, "The Breast Implant Fiasco," *California Law Review*, 87 (1999): 457.

340 Dr. Neal [sic] Rose's Testimony, Trial Transcript at 139, *Johnson v. Bristol-Myers Squibb*: Noel Rose to Docket Management Branch, FDA, September 12, 1990 (letter solicited by Inamed).

341 Despite O'Quinn's jury selection efforts, six men and six women heard the evidence and deliberated their decision. Despite O'Quinn's theories about differing gender attitudes, all six women and four of six men signed the verdict. According to the October 31, 2009, *New York Times*, Mr. O'Quinn died instantly when one of the eight hundred and fifty automobiles in his collection jumped the median of a highway outside Houston, crossed several lanes of traffic and crashed into a tree. He was sixty-eight and not wearing a seat belt.

Chapter 13

342 Alexis de Tocqueville, *Democracy in America*, Vol. I, 18.

343 Laurence J. Peter, *Peter's Quotations: Ideas for our Time* (New York: William Morrow, 1977) 291.

344   Kenneth D. Ackerman, *Dark Horse: The Surprise Election and Political Murder of President James A. Garfield,* (New York: Carroll & Graf, 2003), 443–44. The Guiteau trial proved a showcase for the new specialty of psychiatry, and it highlighted the deficiencies of the M'Naghten rule, holding that defendants could be considered legally insane only if it could be proved that they had failed to understand the consequences of their violent act.

345   "Whale a mammal or a fish" is a paraphrasing of remarks by Henry Miller, MD, formerly an official of the FDA and currently a senior fellow at the Hoover Institution.

346   The ATLA has since renamed itself the American Association for Justice.

347   Lawrence M. Friedman, *Law in America,* (New York: Random House, 2002), 42–45.

348   Today the language of multiple warnings against even the most obvious dangers ("your baby can suffocate from the cellophane wrapped around this product") is found on most consumer product labels including bottled water, the text of package inserts, decals posted at grocery checkout lanes, myriad wall posters, fine print on the television screen, and the surface of rearview mirrors . . . all designed to fulfill the manufacturer's duty to warn.

349   Joseph Nocera, "Dow Corning Succumbs," *Fortune,* October 30, 1995, 137–40.

350   Joseph Goulden, *The Money Lawyers* (New York: Truman Talley, 2006), 156–65.

351   Albert E. Munson et al., "Immunotoxicology of Silicone in Mice," cited in grant submitted to Plastic Surgery Educational Foundation, 1992. Ross Rudolph, Jerrold Abraham, Thomas Vecchione, Seven Guber, Marilyn Woodward, "Myofibroblasts and Free Silicon Around Breast Implants," *Plastic and Reconstructive Surgery* 62 (1978): 185–96.

352   Hans Berkel, Dale C. Birdsell, Heather Jenkins, "Breast Augmentation: A Risk Factor For Breast Cancer?" *New England Journal Medicine* 326 (1992): 1649–53.

353   *Turner vs. Dow Corning Corporation et al.,* Civil Action #92-CV-150, District Court for the City and County of Denver, Colorado, May 24, 1993.

354   Charles Van Devander, "Silicone-trial Verdict Correct, Says Juror," *Rocky Mountain News,* June 18, 1993.

355   Nocera, "Dow Corning Succumbs," 140–42.

356   Ibid., 141.

357   Based on interview with Donald McGhan. Inamed settled for $28 million.

358   Kenneth Feinberg interviewed by the author in 2006.

359   Goulden, *The Money Lawyers,* 171.

360   Ibid., 165.

361   Mark A. Schusterman et al., "Incidence of Autoimmune Disease in Patients after Breast Reconstruction with Silicone Gel Implants Versus Autogenous Tissue: A Preliminary Report," *Annals of Plastic Surgery* 21 (1993): 1–6. Sherine E. Gabriel, et al, "Risk of Connective-Tissue Diseases and Other Disorders after Breast Implantation," *New England Journal of Medicine* 330 (1994): 1697–702. *NEJM* executive editor Marcia Angell was later served a subpoena demanding a deposition to learn why the Mayo Clinic study was published when it was. "Absolutely ridiculous," answered Editor in Chief Jerome Kassirer, "We are in collusion with nobody." When support for the study from the Plastic Surgery Education Foundation was revealed by the *Houston Chronicle,* Kassirer answered for Angell, "The data are the data, no matter what the support is."

362   The abstract was generated from the proceedings of a medical meeting where the Harvard data was first presented and discussed but this was not considered sufficient in a Texas court to serve as peer-reviewed medical evidence.

363   See Fumento.com for February 27, 1996, summary of FDA-imposed injunction of Detecsil.

364   Goulden, *The Money Lawyers,* 165.

365   Nocera, "Dow Corning Succumbs," 154–55.

366   Charles Preuss, attorney representing 3M, interviewed by the author in 2008.

367   *Levine et al. vs. Bristol-Myers Squibb.*

368   The commissioner's declaration is apparently lost to those who maintain the agency's website, which continues to list connective tissue disease a potential risk of breast implantation. See http://www.fda.gov.

369   David A. Kessler testimony before the Subcommittee on Human Resources and Intergovernmental Relations, Committee on Government Reform and Oversight, August 1995. NIH Atypical Rheumatic Diseases and Silicone Breast Implants Workshop held on April 17, 1997.

370   Joseph M. Price and Gretchen Gates Kelly, "Junk Science in the Courtroom: Causes, Effects, and Controls," *Hamline Law Review* 19 (1996): 395–407.

371   Debra L. Worthington et al., "Hindsight Bias, *Daubert*, and the Silicone Breast Implant Litigation: Making the Case for Court-appointed Experts in Complex Medical and Scientific Litigation" *Psychology, Public Policy, and Law* 8 (2002): 154–79.

372   Ibid., 161–63.

373   *Daubert v. Merrell Dow Pharmaceuticals.* 509 US 579 (1993).

374   Karl Popper, *Conjectures and Refutations,* (New York: Basic Books, 1962). Popper famously declared falsifiability to be what distinguishes theories that are scientific from all other theories that are not. Theories framed in such a way that nothing could falsify them were not scientific at all.

375   Bernstein, "The Breast Implant Fiasco," 457–510.

376   Michael E. Reed, "*Daubert* and the Breast Implant Litigation: How is the Judiciary Addressing the Science?" *Plastic and Reconstructive Surgery* 100 (1997): 1322–26.

377   Jorge Sanchez-Guerrero et al., "Silicone Breast Implants and the Risk of Connective-tissue Diseases and Symptoms," *New England Journal of Medicine* 332 (1995) 1666–70. Relative risk is also referred to as the risk ratio. A risk that is one tenth of another risk has a relative risk of 0.1.

378   Laura L. Perkins et al., "A Meta-Analysis of Breast Implants and Connective Tissue Disease," *Annals of Plastic Surgery* 35 (1995): 561–70.

379 *Hall v. Baxter Healthcare Corp.*, 947 F. Supp. 1387 (D. Or. 1996)

380 *In re* Breast Implant Cases, 942 F. Supp. 958, 960 (E. & S. D. N. Y., 1996). Betty A. Diamond, "Silicone Breast Implants in Relation to Connective Tissue Diseases and Immunologic Dysfunction," A Report by a National Science Panel to the Hon. Sam D. Pointer Jr., Coordinating Judge for the Federal Breast Implant Multi-District Litigation, November 17, 1998. A. Manning, "Breast-implant plaintiffs claim bias negates study," *USA Today*, April 14, 1999.

381 Barbara S. Hulka, "Experience of a Science Panel Formed to Advise the Federal Judiciary on Silicone Breast Implants," *New England Journal of Medicine*, March 16, 2000.

382 Independent Review Group: Report on Silicone Gel Breast Implants (1998), available at http://www.silicone-review. gov.uk/silicone/index.htm.

383 Institute of Medicine, *Safety of Breast Implants* (1999). Whereas the FDA had chosen to ignore the immunotoxicity studies of Kimber White, the IOM panel was grateful for his testimony, which amounted to a clean bill of immunologic health for the silicone polymers used in medical devices.

384 While the IOM was able to complete its review and reach final conclusions, the FDA had also completed its own "epidemiologic review" led by two outspoken critics of breast implants, Lori Brown and Barbara Silverman. Although each held MPH degrees and presumably enjoyed some expertise with epidemiologic methods, they were unable to agree that enough studies had been completed to rule out a "moderately increased risk" of connective tissue disease. Dr. Kessler added his name to the list of coauthors. See Barbara G. Silverman et al., "Reported Complications of Silicone Gel Breast Implants: An Epidemiologic Review," *Archives of Internal Medicine*, 124 (1996): 744–56.

385 Martha Grigg, Stuart Bondurant et al., *Information for Women About the Safety of Silicone Breast Implants*, (Washington, DC: National Academy Press, June 22, 1999).

386 As of this writing, October 15, 2014, the FDA website continues to list connective tissue disease as a risk of breast
implantation, stating, "In order to rule out these complications, studies would have to be larger and longer than those
conducted so far."

Chapter 14

387 Alexander Hamilton, James Madison, John Jay, *The Federalist,* 1788.

388 Johan Norberg, "Humanity's Greatest Achievement," *Wall
Street Journal,* October 2, 2006.

389 As late as November 1990, ASPRS released a survey of
592 women, 93 percent of whom reported they were fully
satisfied with their breast implants, 96 percent of whom
would have the surgery again. Left unexplained was what
the other 4 percent were thinking and why. The data were
largely ignored by the press and meant little to the FDA and
committees of Congress.

390 Jon Kent, ASPRS lobbyist, reporting conversation with Senator Hatch, February 23, 1994. Dr. Edwards spoke directly
to the author. James Benson's reflections transcribed
from conversation with Garry Brody on April 11, 1994. If
Dr. Kessler did in fact read the entire Dow Corning PMA
(fifty thousand pages) he should have noted immunotoxity
studies, case control studies, and opinions from recognized
authorities, all of it disregarded by trial attorneys, activists,
and his agency alike.

391 Orrin Hatch, *Square Peg: Confessions of a Citizen Senator,* (New York: Basic Books, 2002), 81–89. "Snake Oil:
Regulating Food Supplements," *The Economist,* February
7, 2004. Jane Brody, "Potential for Harm in Dietary Supplements," *New York Times,* April 8, 2008. "Time to Ban
Ephedra," *Wall Street Journal,* April 20, 2005. Penni Crabtree, "Little Pill, Big Trouble," *San Diego Union-Tribune,* July
20, 2003. Penni Crabtree, "Metabolife Loses: Must pay
$7.46 million," *San Diego Union-Tribune,* June 24, 2004

(supplement manufacturers were protected from regulation but not from civil litigation arising from bodily injury).

392   Chris Adams, "FDA Isn't Holding Up in Court: Agency's Credibility Falters Due to Batch of Notable Losses," *Wall Street Journal*, November 19, 2002.

393   The Center for Biologics Evaluation and Research, which is funded for research in the development of vaccines and blood products, is a noteworthy exception.

394   Error distinctions frequently highlighted by Hoover fellow and former FDA Director of Biotechnology Henry Miller, MD.

395   Critics of EMA argue that with speed of review comes a greater chance of postmarket safety withdrawals. For a determination that there were no differences in safety withdrawals between the US, UK, and Spain, see O. M. Bakke et al., "Drug Safety Discontinuations in the United Kingdom, United States, and Spain from 1974 through 1993: A Regulatory Perspective," *Clinical Pharmacology and Therapeutics* 58 (1995): 108–117.

396   "Kessler Crew Lobbying Clinton For Retention," *Food & Drug Insider Report*, November 30, 1992. Henry I. Miller, "At FDA, Kessler Leaves a Negative Legacy," *New York Times*, December 1, 1996.

397   John Solomon, "FDA Chief's Expenses Questioned in Review," *Associated Press* as reported in *Pasadena Star-News*, November 2, 1996. "Ex-FDA Chief Moves to Yale," *Associated Press*, February 13, 1997, in which Yale University President Richard C. Levin is quoted lauding Kessler as the most distinguished commissioner the agency ever had.

398   Marcia Angell, *Science on Trial: The Clash of Medical Evidence and the Law in the Breast Implant Case,"* (New York: W. W. Norton, 1996). Alternative or integrative or complementary medicine (CAM) accounts for expenditures in excess of $47 billion each year, at least forty states license CAM providers, and institutions such as Johns Hopkins Hospital and Sloan Kettering Cancer Center incorporate programs such as

aromatherapy. "The Touch That Doesn't Heal," *Wall Street Journal,*" December 28, 2008.

399   Under conditional fees, the lawyer receives a premium only if the case is won and nothing if the case is lost. The premium is both in theory and often in practice unrelated to the damage award.

400   Angell, *Science on Trial.* Bernstein, "The Breast Implant Fiasco," 457–510.

401   These studies all cited in earlier chapters. Dow Corning's chemist Robert Levier reported to the FDA rates of gel bleed depending on implant barrier shield that ranged from .096 grams to .48 grams per year. Taken as an average of .288 grams, this represents one/hundredth of an ounce.

402   Study of Trilucent soybean oil-filled implant approved by FDA on July 15, 1994. Jack C. Fisher, "Vegetable Oil Implant? That's Junk Doctor!" Letter to the Editor, *Wall Street Journal,* February 1994. The author also wrote to Sidney Wolfe (without response) to describe his personal experience treating mentally ill patients with wounds resulting from self-injected vegetable oils that produced inflammatory reactions not easily resolved. Stanley Monstrey, A. Christophe, J. Delanghe, S. De Vriese, M. Hamdi, K. Van Landuyt, and P. Blondeel, "What Exactly Was Wrong with the Trilucent Breast Implants? A Unifying Hypothesis," *Plastic & Reconstructive Surgery,* March 2004, 847–56.

403   See http://www.fda.gov for log of drugs and devices reviewed and approved according to year. See also risks still listed for breast implants, including connective tissue diseases.

404   "Implants and Science," *Wall Street Journal,* November 20, 2006.

405   Sheryl Gay Stolberg, "Botox Commercials Mislead Consumers, Government Says," *New York Times,* September 11, 2002.

406   Thomas Stossel, "Witch Hunt," *Wall Street Journal,* February 21, 2006. Thomas Stossel, "Regulation of Financial Conflicts

of Interest in Medical Practice and Medical Research: A Damaging Solution in Search of a Problem," *Perspectives in Biology & Medicine* 50 (July 31, 2007): 54–71.

407 Thomas Stossel and David Shaywitz, "What's Wrong With Money in Science?" *Washington Post,* July 2, 2006.

408 As of this writing in October 2014, headlines such as "Doctors Net Billions from Drug Firms" (*Wall Street Journal,* October 1, 2014) draw attention to data collected in compliance with the "Sunshine Clause" of the ACA that cannot yet distinguish between a gift of bagels and payment of a contract obligation.

409 Alexander Hamilton, John Jay, James Madison, *The Federalist,* 1788, (#51 written by James Madison).

Epilogue

410 Andrew Wood, "Dow Corning Starting a New Chapter," *Chemical Week,* August 11, 2004.

411 The number of consecutive studies showing no causal link between silicone and any rheumatic, autoimmune, connective tissue, or other disease now exceeds thirty.

412 David Shepardson, "Court extends Dow Corning breast implant settlement to 'tissue expanders,' " *Detroit News,* July 31, 2014.

413 Matt Blunt, "How Missouri Cut Junk Lawsuits," *Wall Street Journal,* September 22, 2009. "Loser Pays, Everybody Wins," *Wall Street Journal,* December 15, 2010.

414 "Wal-Mart's Class Victory," *Wall Street Journal,* June 21, 2011. L. Gordon Crovitz, "The Supreme Court and the Tyranny of Lawyers," *Wall Street Journal,* March 9, 2009.

415 Henry Miller, personal communication.

416 Evan Bayh, "ObamaCare's Tax Raid on Medical Devices," *Wall Street Journal,* September 28, 2012. Henry Miller, "ObamaCare's Killer Device Tax," *Wall Street Journal,* May 11, 2012. Henry Miller, "FDA Has Device Makers Looking Outside U. S.," *OCRegister.com,* July 18, 2012. As of this writing, the United States already maintains the highest corporate

tax rate in the developed world, to which a medical device excise tax on sales and the most restrictive regulatory apparatus combine to threaten a steady loss of this industry to other nations.

417　Platinum toxicity promoted by the nonprofit group Chemically Associated Neurologic Disorders. Joseph K. McLaughlin et al., "Long Term Cancer Risk Among Swedish Women With Cosmetic Breast Implants: Update of a Nationwide Study," *Journal of the National Cancer Institute* 98 (2006): 557–60. A plausible explanation for the decrease is the tumor sparing effect of hypothermia. Like the hypothermic testicle in its scrotum, the breast gland displaced by a silicone implant exists at about two degrees lower than normal body temperature.

418　"Prescription for the FDA," *Wall Street Journal*, July 19, 2002. Henry Miller, "Can Dr. McClellan Cure the FDA?" *Hoover Digest*, 2004 No. 1. Political scientist Francis Fukuyama suggests that we now live in a vetocracy instead of democracy. See his *Political Order and Political Decay*. See http://www.fda.gov under past commissioners for terms of duty and gaps between.

419　Lauran Neergard, "Eased FDA Rules on Food Labels Draw Opposition," *Associated Press*, October 20, 2002.

420　Henry Miller, "Lackadaisical FDA Needs a Dose of Vitality from a New Chief," *Los Angeles Times*, March 1, 2004.

421　The author visited the history office and wishes to thank historian Suzanne Junod for her assistance, also for a copy of her doctoral thesis, "Chemistry and Controversy: Regulating the Use of Chemicals in Foods, 1883–1959," Emory University, 1994. Tufts University Center for the Study of Drug Development monitors and reports both the speed and the costs of new drug approvals. See http://www.fda.gov for annual budget itemization.

422　Andrew von Eschenbach, "Medical Innovation: How the US Can Retain Its Lead," *Wall Street Journal*, February 14, 2012, Henry I. Miller, *To America's Health: A Proposal to*

Reform the Food and Drug Administration, (Stanford, CA: Hoover Institution Press: 2000). Henry Miller, "Wrong Rx for the FDA," *Los Angeles Times,* March 5, 2012.

423 Alicia Mundy, "A Wolfe in Regulator's Clothing: Drug Industry Critic Joins FDA," *WSJ.com,* January 6, 2004.

424 John A. Keech and Brevator J. Creech, "Anaplastic T-Cell Lymphoma in Proximity to a Saline-Filled Breast Implant," *Plastic Reconstructive Surgery,* 100 (1997): 554–55. Garry S. Brody, Dennis Deapen, et al., "Anaplastic Large Cell Lymphoma (ALCL) Occurring in Women With Breast Implants: Analysis of 173 Cases," in press (due March, 2015).

425 See http://www.citizen.org. For his plastic surgeon cover-up theory, Dr. Wolfe features the careless remark of a single plastic surgeon and ignores the FDA liaison with ASPS and its close monitoring of ALCL.

426 The Center for Devices and Radiological Health, U. S. Food and Drug Administration, "Anaplastic Large Cell Lymphoma (ALCL) in Women with Breast Implants Preliminary FDA Findings and Analysis," January 2011. Their designation "breast ALCL" is misleading because these tumors clearly arise in the fibrous sheath that surrounds the implant that lies behind the breast gland.

427 McLaughlin's study of Swedish women (see footnote 8 in Epilogue) cites nineteen fewer cancers among 3,486 women followed for an average of 18.4 years.

428 Statistics maintained and reported by the American Society of Plastic Surgery (http://plasticsurgery.org). Three hundred thousand represents 20 percent of 15 million cosmetic procedures, 14 percent of 21 million total plastic surgery procedures (2013). Jennifer L. Baker, Brian Mailey, Christopher A. Tokin, Sarah L. Blair, Anne M. Wallace, "Postmastectomy Reconstruction Is Associated with Improved Survival in Patients with Invasive Breast Cancer: A Single-Institution Study," *American Surgery* 79 (2013): 977–81.

429 John Adams, Argument in defense of the Soldiers in the Boston Massacre Trials, December 1770.

430 American Council on Science and Health (http://www.
     acsh.org) offers numerous examples of the precautionary
     principle as it is frequently misapplied.
431 Refers to Rachel Carson's *Silent Spring*, an all-time junk sci-
     ence classic.

BIBLIOGRAPHY

Adams, Francis. *The Genuine Works of Hippocrates*. Baltimore: Williams & Wilkins, 1939.

Allen, Frederick. *Secret Formula*. New York: Harper Collins, 1994.

Ames, Bruce N., and Lois Swirsky Gold. "Chemical Carcinogenesis: Too Many Rodent Carcinogens." *Proceedings of the National Academy of Sciences* 87 (1990): 7772–76.

Ames, Bruce N., Margie Profet, and Lois Swirsky Gold. "Nature's Chemicals and Synthetic Chemicals: Comparative Toxicology." *Proceedings of the National Academy of Sciences* 87 (1990): 7782–85.

Angell, Marcia. "Breast Implants—Protection or Paternalism." *New England Journal of Medicine* 326 (1992): 1695–96.

Angell, Marcia. *Science on Trial: The Clash of Medical Evidence and the Law in the Breast Implant Case*. New York: W. W. Norton, 1996.

Arion, H. G. "Prosthesis Retromammaires," *Comptes Rendus de la Société Francaises de Gynécologie* 35: 427–31, 1965.

Ashley, Frank L. "A New Type of Breast Prosthesis: Preliminary Report." *Plastic Reconstructive Surgery* 45 (1970): 45.

Baker, James L. "Augmentation Mammaplasty." In J. Q. Owsley and R. A. Peterson, *Symposium on Aesthetic Surgery of the Breast*. St. Louis: C. V. Mosby, 1978, 256–63.

Baker, James L., Roger J. Bartels, and William M. Douglas. "Closed Compression for Rupturing a Contracted Capsule Around a Breast Implant." *Plastic Reconstructive Surgery* 58 (1976): 137–41.

Baker, Jennifer L., Brian Mailey, Christopher A. Tokin, Sarah L. Blair, Anne M. Wallace. "Postmastectomy Reconstruction Is Associated with Improved Survival in Patients with Invasive Breast Cancer: A Single-Institution Study." *American Surgery* 79 (2013): 977–81.

Bakke, O. M., M. A. Manocchia, F. de Abajo, K. I. Kaitin, and L. Lasagna. "Drug Safety Discontinuations in the United Kingdom, United States, and Spain from 1974 through 1993: A Regulatory Perspective." *Clinical Pharmacology and Therapeutics* 58 (1995): 108–117.

Balkin, S. W. "The Fluid Silicone Prosthesis." *Symposium on Implants in Foot Surgery: Clinics in Podiatry* 1 (1984): 145–64.

Balkin, S. W., and L. Kaplan. "Injectable Silicone and the Diabetic Foot: A 25-Year Report," *The Foot* 1 (July 1991): 83–88.

Beisang, Arthur A., Richard A. Geise, and Robert A. Ersek. "A Radiolucent Prosthetic Gel." *Plastic and Reconstructive Surgery.* 87 (1991) 855–92.

Benavent, W. J. "Treatment of Bilateral Breast Carcinomas in a Patient with Silicone Gel Breast Implants: Case Report." *Plastic Reconstructive Surgery* 51 (1973): 588.

Benjamin, Ludy T., Anne M. Rogers, and Angela Rosenbaum. "Coca-Cola, Caffeine, and Mental Deficiency: Harry Hollingworth and the Chattanooga Trial of 1911." *Journal of the History of Behavioral Sciences,* 27 (1991): 42–55.

Berkel, Hans, Dale C. Birdsell, and Heather Jenkins. "Breast Augmentation: A Risk Factor For Breast Cancer?" *New England Journal of Medicine* 326 (1992): 1649–53.

Bernstein, David E. "The Breast Implant Fiasco." *California Law Review* 87 (1999): 457–510.

Bernstein, Michael A. *A Perilous Progress: Economists and Public Purpose in the Twentieth Century.* Princeton, NJ: Princeton University Press, 2001.

Bernstein, Peter L. *Against the Gods: The Remarkable Story of Risk.* New York: John Wiley & Sons, 1996.

Berscheid, Ellen, and Elaine Walster. "Physical Attractiveness." *Advances in Experimental Social Psychology* 7 (1974): 157–205.

Berscheid, Ellen, and Steve Gangestad. "The Social Psychological Implications of Facial Physical Attractiveness." *Clinics in Plastic Surgery* 9 (1982): 289–96.

Biggs, Thomas M., Jean Cukier, and L. Fabian Worthing. "Augmentation Mammaplasty: A Review of 18 Years." *Plastic Reconstructive Surgery* 69 (1982): 445–50.

Boorstin, Daniel. *The Americans: The Democratic Experience.* New York: Vintage Books, 1973.

Bower, D. G., and C. B. Radlauer. "Breast Cancer after Prophylactic Subcutaneous Mastectomies and Reconstruction with Silastic Prosthesis." *Plastic Reconstructive Surgery* 44 (1969): 541.

Braley, Silas A. "The Use of Silicones in Plastic Surgery, A Retrospective View." *Plastic and Reconstructive Surgery* 51 (1973) 280–288.

Brand, K. Gerhard. "Diversity and Complexity of Carcinogenic Processes: Conceptual Inferences from Foreign-Body Tumorigenesis." *Journal of the National Cancer Institute* 57 (1976): 973–76.

Breo, Dennis L. "Sidney Wolfe, MD—Healing the System or Just Raising Hell?" *Journal of the American Medical Association* 266 (1991): 1131–33.

Brinkley, Alan. *The End of Reform: New Deal Liberalism in Recession and War.* New York: Alfred A. Knopf, 1995.

Brody, Garry S. "Fact and Fiction about Breast Implant "Bleed." *Plastic and Reconstructive Surgery* 60 (1977): 615–16.

Brody, Garry S., Dennis Deapen, C. R. Taylor, L. Pinter-Brown, S. R. House-Lightner, J. Andersen, G. Carlson, G. M. Lechner, and E. Alan. "Anaplastic Large Cell Lymphoma (ALCL) Occurring in Women With Breast Implants: Analysis of 173 Cases." In press (due March 2015).

Burkhardt, Boyd R. "Comparing Contracture Rates: Probability Theory and the Unilateral Contracture." *Plastic and Reconstructive Surgery* 74 (1984): 527–29.

Byrne, John A. *Informed Consent.* New York: McGraw Hill, 1996.

Cancer Facts and Figures 2004. American Cancer Society, New York, 2004. http://www.pink-ribbon-pins.com/CancerRates2004.pdf

Candler, Charles Howard. *Asa Griggs Candler.* Atlanta: Emory University Press.

Candler, Charles Howard. "The True Origins of Coca-Cola." Coca-Cola Miscellany: Special Collections, Woodruff Library, Emory University.

Cardy, Richard H. "Carcinogenicity and Chronic Toxicity of 2,4-Toluenediamine in Fischer 344 Rats." *Journal of the National Cancer Institute* 62 (1979): 1107–16.

Caro, Robert. *The Years of Lyndon Johnson: Master of the Senate.* New York: Alfred Knopf, 2002.

Colebrook, Leonard and Meave Kenny. "Treatment of Human Puerperal Infections, and of Experimental Infections in Mice, with Prontosil." *Lancet* 1 (1936): 1279–86.

Coppin, Clayton, and Jack High. *Politics of Purity: Harvey Washington Wiley and the Origins of Federal Food Policy.* Ann Arbor: University of Michigan Press, 1999.

Cronin, Thomas D., and Frank J. Gerow. "Augmentation Mammaplasty: A New 'Natural Feel' Prosthesis." *Excerpta Medica International Congress* 66 (1963): 41–49.

Cronin, Thomas D., and Roger L. Greenberg. "Our Experience with the Silastic Gel Breast Prosthesis." In *Plastic and Reconstructive Surgery,* 46 (1970): 1–7.

Deapen, Dennis M. "Breast Cancer and Augmentation Mammaplasty." *Conference Proceedings: Silicone in Medical Devices.* Center for Devices and Radiologic Health: FDA, December 1991.

Deapen, Dennis M., Malcolm C. Pike, John T. Casagrande, and Garry S. Brody. "The Relationship between Breast Cancer and Augmentation Mammaplasty: An Epidemiologic Study." *Plastic Reconstructive Surgery* 77 (1986): 361–67.

"Deaths Following Elixir of Sulfanilamide-Massengill." *Journal of the American Medical Association* 109 (1937): 1367.

DeNicola, R. Robert. "Permanent Artificial (Silicone) Urethra." *Journal of Urology,* 63 (1950): 168–72.

de Tocqueville, Alexis. *Democracy in America,* Volume I.

DiConti, Veronica D. "The Federal Trade Commission." In George T. Kurian, *A Historical Guide to the U. S. Government.* Oxford: Oxford University Press, 1998.

Dodson, J. Lynne. *"A Century of Oncology."* Greenwich, CT: Greenwich Press, 1997.

Doll, Richard. "Cohort Studies: History of the Method, 1. Prospective Cohort Studies." *Soz Präventivmed* 46 (2001): 75–86.

Doll, Richard. "Cohort Studies: History of the Method, 2. Retrospective Cohort Studies." *Soz Präventivmed* 46 (2001): 152–60.

Dowling Harry, *Magic in a Bottle*. New York: Appleton-Century, 1943.

"Dr. Wiley's Resignation." *Scientific American*, March 30, 1912, 282.

Edward, Charles A. *Tough Choices: My Extraordinary Journey at the Heart of American Politics and Medicine*. Privately published, 2005.

Estrin N. F., and James M. Akerson. *Cosmetic Regulation in a Competitive Environment*. New York: Marcel Dekker, 2000.

Etcoff, Nancy. *Survival of the Prettiest: The Science of Beauty*. New York: Anchor Books, 2000.

"Excerpts and Summary of a National Conference on Medical Devices." *Journal of the American Medical Association* 210 (1969): 1745.

Fernandez-Armesto, Felipe. *Near a Thousand Tables: A History of Food*. New York: The Free Press, 2002.

Festing, Michael F. W., and Elizabeth M. C. Fisher. "Mighty Mice." *Nature* 404 (2000): 815.

Fisher, Alan C., and Wendy Worth. Revised by Debra A. Mayer. *Is There a Cancer Epidemic in the United States?* American Council on Science and Health, 1995.

Fisher, Jack C. "The Silicone Controversy: When Will Science Prevail?" *New England Journal of Medicine* 326 (1992) 1696–1698.

Frankel, Alison. "From Pioneers to Profits: The Splendid Past and the Muddled Present of Breast Implant Litigation." *The American Lawyer* (June 1992): 82–91.

Friedman, Lawrence M. *Law in America*. New York: Random House, 2002.

Gabriel, Sherine E., W. Michael O'Fallon, Leonard T. Kurland, C. Mary Beard, John E. Woods, and L. Joseph Melton. "Risk of Connective-Tissue Diseases and Other Disorders after Breast Implantation." *New England Journal of Medicine* 330 (1994): 1697–702.

Gage, Andrew. "The Development of the Implantable Cardiac Pacemaker." In *Medical History in Buffalo 1846–1996: Collected Essays*, edited by Lilli Sentz 247–56. Buffalo, NY: History of Medicine Collection, State University of New York–Buffalo, 1996.

Gayou, Robert, and Ross Rudolph. "Capsular Contraction Around Silicone Mammary Prostheses." *Annals Plastic Surgery* 2 (1979): 62–71.

Goin, John M., and Marcia Kraft Goin. *Changing the Body: Psychological Effects of Plastic Surgery.* Baltimore: Williams & Wilkins, 1981.

Goldwyn, Robert M. *The Patient and the Plastic Surgeon.* Boston: Little Brown & Co., 1991.

Goldwyn, Robert M. "Vincenz Czerny and the Beginnings of Breast Reconstruction." *Plastic and Reconstructive Surgery* 61 (1978): 673–81.

Gonzalez-Ulloa, Mario. *The Creation of Aesthetic Plastic Surgery.* New York: Springer-Verlag, 1976.

Goulden, Joseph. *The Money Lawyers.* New York: Truman Talley, 2006.

Grant, Nicole J. *The Selling of Contraception: The Dalkon Shield Case, Sexuality, and Women's Autonomy.* Columbus: Ohio State University Press, 1992.

Grigg, Martha, Stuart Bondurant, Virginia L. Ernster and Roger Herdman. *Information for Women About the Safety of Silicone Breast Implants.* Washington, DC: National Academy Press, June 22, 1999.

Halberstam, David. *The Fifties.* New York: Villard Books, 1993.

Hamilton, Alexander, James Madison, and John Jay. *The Federalist.* 1788.

Hargreaves, Mary W. M. "The Durum Wheat Controversy." *Agricultural History,* 42 (1968) 211–229.

Hatch, Orrin. *Square Peg: Confessions of a Citizen Senator.* New York: Basic Books, 2002.

Havender, William R. "The Science and Politics of Cyclamate." *The Public Interest* 71 (1983): 17–31.

Hawkins, Mary F. *Unshielded: The Human Cost of the Dalkon Shield.* Toronto: University of Toronto Press, 1997.

Hayes, Harry. *An Anthology of Plastic Surgery.* Rockville, MD: Aspen, 1986.

Hazlitt, William. *Lectures on the English Comic Writers.* New York: Wiley and Putnam, 1845.

Hester, T. Roderick, F. Nahai, J. Bostwick, and J. Cukic. "A Five-Year Experience with Polyurethane-Covered Mammary Prostheses for Treatment of Capsular Contracture, Primary Augmentation Mammoplasty, and Breast Reconstruction." *Clinics in Plastic Surgery* 15 (1988): 569–85.

Hilts, Philip J. *Protecting America's Health: The FDA, Business, and One Hundred Years of Regulation.* New York: Alfred Knopf, 2003.

"History of ASPRS." *Plastic and Reconstructive Surgery* 94 (September 1994) 72A–73A.

Hollingworth, H. L. "The Influence of Caffein on Mental and Motor Efficiency." *Archives of Psychology* 22 (1912): iii.

Holstein, Jean. *The First Fifty Years at The Jackson Laboratory.* Bar Harbor, ME: The Jackson Laboratory, 1979.

Hoopes, John E., Milton T. Edgerton, and William Shelley. "Organic Synthetics and Augmentation Mammaplasty: Their Relation to Breast Cancer." *Plastic Reconstructive Surgery* 39 (1967): 263–69.

Hulka, Barbara S., Nancy L. Kerkvliet, and Peter Tugwell. "Experience of a Science Panel Formed to Advise the Federal Judiciary on Silicone Breast Implants." *New England Journal of Medicine* 1, 342 (2000): 812–15.

Hutt, Peter Barton. "Enactment of the 1958 Delaney Clause." In *Food and Drug Law: Cases and Materials.* 868–72. Westbury, NY: The Foundation Press, 1991.

Hutt, Peter Barton. "A History of Government Regulation of Adulteration and Misbranding of Food." *Food, Drug, Cosmetic Law Journal* 39 (1984): 2–5.

Hutt, Peter Barton. "A History of Government Regulation of Adulteration and Misbranding of Medical Devices." *Food, Drug, Cosmetic Law Journal* 44 (1989): 99–105.

Hutt, Peter Barton. "The Transformation of United States Food and Drug Law." *Journal of the Association of Food & Drug Officials* 60 (1996): 1–62.

Jackson, Charles O. *Food and Drug Legislation in the New Deal.* Princeton, NJ: Princeton University Press, 1970.

Jefferson, Thomas. *Notes on Virginia.* Query XVII, 1781–1785.

Johnson, Paul. *A History of the American People.* New York: HarperCollins, 1997.

Junod, Suzanne. "Chemistry and Controversy: Regulating the Use of Chemicals in Foods, 1883–1959." PhD diss, Emory University, 1994.

Junod, Suzanne White. "Harvey Wiley: His Life and Times." *The Food and Drug Law Institute Update.* June 2000 (http://www.fdli.org).

Kagan, H. D. "Sakurai Injectable Silicone Formula." *Archives of Otolaryngology* 78 (1962): 663.

Keech, John A., and Brevator J. Creech. "Anaplastic T-Cell Lymphoma in Proximity to a Saline-Filled Breast Implant." *Plastic Reconstructive Surgery,* 100 (1997): 554–55.

Kelsey, Frances O. "Thalidomide Update: Regulatory Aspects." *Teratology* 38 (1988): 221–26.

Kerrigan, Carolyn L. *Report on the Meme Breast Implant: Prepared for the Minister of Health and Welfare Canada.* Montreal: Division of Plastic Surgery, McGill University, 1989.

Kessler, David. "The Basis for the FDA's Decision on Breast Implants." *New England Journal of Medicine* 326 (1992): 1713–15.

Kessler, David. *A Question of Intent: A Great American Battle with a Deadly Industry.* New York: Public Affairs/Perseus Books Group, 2001.

Kiskadden, W. S. "Operations on Bosoms Dangerous." *Plastic Reconstructive Surgery* 15 (1955): 79.

Kolko, Gabriel. *Triumph of Conservatism.* New York: Free Press of Glencoe, 1964.

Kondo, Hirobumi, Yasuo Kumagai, Yuichi Shiokawa. "Scleroderma Following Cosmetic Surgery ("Adjuvant Disease"): A Review of Nine Cases Reported in Japan." In *Current Topics in Rheumatology: Systemic Sclerosis (Scleroderma).* New York: Gower Publishing Company Ltd., 1981, 135–37.

Kumagai, Yasuo, Abe Chiyuki, and Yuchi Shiokawa. "Scleroderma After Cosmetic Surgery: Four Cases of Human Adjuvant Disease." *Arthritis and Rheumatism* 22 (1979): 532–37.

Lalardrie, J. P., and R. Mouly. "History of Mammaplasty." In Gonzalez-Ulloa, *The Creation of Aesthetic Plastic Surgery*, New York: Springer-Verlag, 1976, 135–44.

Lieberman, Adam J. "Love Canal, 1978." In *Facts Versus Fears*, Publication of the American Council on Science and Health, 1997, 14–15.

Liebhafsky, Herman A. *Silicones under the Monogram: A Story of Industrial Research*. New York: John Wiley & Sons, 1978.

London, William H. "60 Minutes on Health: Picks and Pans." http://www.acsh.org, January 1, 2000.

London, William M., and John W. Morgan. "Living Long Enough to Die of Cancer." *Priorities* 7 (1995): 6–9.

Long, Perrin H. *Journal of the American Medical Association* 108 (1937): 32–37.

Maher, Brendan A. "Test Tubes With Tails." *The Scientist* 16 (2002): 22–24.

Marchant, June. "Breast Prostheses." *Lancet* 2 (1975): 187–88.

McDowell, Frank. "James Barrett Brown, Obituary." *Plastic and Reconstructive Surgery* 48 (1971): 101–4.

McFayden, Richard E. "Thalidomide in America: A Brush with Tragedy." *Clio Medica* 11 (1976): 79–93.

McLaughlin, Joseph K., Loren Lipworth, Jon P. Fryzek, Weimin Ye, Robert E. Tarone, and Olof Nyren. "Long Term Cancer Risk Among Swedish Women With Cosmetic Breast Implants: Update of a Nationwide Study." *Journal of the National Cancer Institute* 98 (2006): 557–60.

Miller, Henry I. "Can Dr. McClellan Cure the FDA?" *Hoover Digest*, 1 (2004).

Miller, Henry I. *To America's Health: A Proposal to Reform the Food and Drug Administration*. Stanford, CA: Hoover Institution Press: 2000.

Mintz, Morton. *By Prescription Only*. Boston: Beacon Press, 1967.

Mishra, Nirmal K. "Hypothesis for a Potential Mechanism of Silicone-Induced Carcinogenesis." *Conference Proceedings: Silicone in Medical Devices*. Center for Devices and Radiologic Health: FDA, December 1991, 155–68.

Moeller, Susan D. *Compassion Fatigue: How the Media Sell Disease, Famine, War, and Death.* New York City: Routledge, 1999.

Monstrey, Stanley, Armand Christophe, Joris Delanghe, Stephanie De Vriese, Moustapha Hamdi, Koenraad M. Van Landuyt, Phillip Blondeel. "What Exactly Was Wrong with the Trilucent Breast Implants? A Unifying Hypothesis." *Plastic & Reconstructive Surgery* 113 (March 2004): 847–56.

Miyoshi, K., T. Miyamura, Y. Kobayashi, T. Itakura, K. Nishijo, M. Higashibara, H. Shiragami, and F. Ohno. "Hypergammaglobuilinemia by Prolonged Adjuvanticity in Man: Disorders Developed after Augmentation Mammaplasty." *Ijishimpo (Japan Medical Journal)* 2112 (1964): 9–14.

Napier, Kristine. "Reworking the Delaney Clause," *Priorities* (Spring 1992): 42–44.

Natenberg, Maurice. *The Legacy of Doctor Wiley and the Administration of his Food and Drug Act.* Chicago: Regent House, 1957.

Newberg, Herbert B. *Newberg on Class Actions.* New York: McGraw-Hill, 1992.

Oppenheimer, B. S., Enid T. Oppenheimer, and Arthur Purdy Stout. "Sarcomas Induced in Rats by Implanting Cellophane." *Proceedings of the Society of Experimental Biology & Medicine* 67 (1948): 33–34.

Oppenheimer, B. S., Enid T. Oppenheimer, Arthur Purdy Stout, and I. Danishefsk. "Malignant Tumors Resulting from Imbedding Plastics in Rodents." *Science* 118 (1953): 305–6.

Oppenheimer, B. S., Enid T. Oppenheimer, I. Danishefsk, Arthur Purdy Stout, and Frederick R. Eirich. "Further Studies of Polymers as Carcinogenic Agents in Animals." *Cancer Research* 15 (1955): 333–40.

Pachter, Henry M. *Magic into Science: The Story of Paracelsus.* New York: Henry Schuman, 1951.

Paneth, Nigel, Ezra Susser, and Mervyn Susser. "Origins and Early Development of the Case-Control Study: Part 1, Early Evolution." *Soz Präventivmed* 47 (2002): 282–88.

Paneth, Nigel, Ezra Susser, and Mervyn Susser. "Origins and Early Development of the Case-Control Study: Part 2, The

Case-Control Study from Lane-Claypon to 1950." *Soz Präventivmed* 47 (2002): 359–65.

Pearse, Herman E. "Results from Using Vitallium Tubes in Biliary Surgery." *Annals of Surgery*, 124 (1946): 1020–1029.

Pendergrast, Mark. *For God, Country, and Coca-Cola.* New York: Macmillan, 1993.

Pennisi, Vincent R. "Long-Term Use of Polyurethane Breast Prostheses: A 14-Year Experience." *Plastic Reconstructive Surgery* 86 (1990): 368–71.

Perkins, Laura L., Brian D. Clark, Patti J. Klein, and Ralph R. Cook. "A Meta-Analysis of Breast Implants and Connective Tissue Disease." *Annals of Plastic Surgery* 35 (1995): 561–70.

Perry, Susan, and Jim Dawson. *Nightmare: Women and the Dalkon Shield.* New York: Macmillan, 1985.

Peter, Lawrence J. *Peter's Quotations: Ideas for our Time.* New York: William Morrow, 1977.

Plaut, Gunther W. *The Torah: A Modern Commentary.* New York: Union of American Hebrew Congregations, 1981.

Pliny. *Natural History,* volume I–X.

Popper, Karl. *Conjectures and Refutations.* New York: Basic Books, 1962.

Postrel Virginia. "Of Mice and Men: Finding Cancer's Causes." *Reason* (December 1991): 18–21.

Prentiss, Robert J., D. C. Boatwright, and R. D. Pennington, W. F. Hohn, and M. H. Schwartz. "Testicular Prosthesis: Materials, Methods, and Results." *Journal of Urology,* 90 (1963): 208–9.

Price, Joseph M., and Gretchen Gates Kelly. "Junk Science in the Courtroom: Causes, Effects, and Controls." *Hamline Law Review* 19 (1996): 395–407.

Raso, Jack. "Nutrition-Related 'Credentialing' Organizations: The Good, the Bad, and the Abysmal. *Priorities* 7 (1999): 31–34.

Reed, Michael E. "*Daubert* and the Breast Implant Litigation: How is the Judiciary Addressing the Science?" *Plastic and Reconstructive Surgery* 100 (1997): 1322–26.

Rosenberg, Lynn. Discussion of "The Relationship Between Breast Cancer and Augmentation Mammaplasty: An Epidemiologic Study." *Plastic Reconstructive Surgery* 77 (1986): 368.

Rowe, Verald K., H. C. Spencer, S. L. Bass. "Toxicological Studies on Certain Commercial Silicones." *Journal of Industrial Hygiene and Toxicology* 30 (1948): 337–52.

Rudolph, Ross, Jerrold Abraham, Thomas Vecchione, Seven Guber, and Marilyn Woodward. "Myofibroblasts and Free Silicon Around Breast Implants." *Plastic and Reconstructive Surgery* 62 (1978): 185–96.

Rudolph, Ross, Jerrold Abraham, Thomas Vecchione, Seven Guber, and Marilyn Woodward. "Myofibroblasts and Free Silicon Around Breast Implants." *Plastic and Reconstructive Surgery* 62 (1978): 185–96.

Rudolph, Ross, Joe Utley, and Marilyn Woodward. "Contractile Fibroblasts in a Painful Pacemaker Pocket." *Annals of Thoracic Surgery* 31 (1981): 373–76.

Sanchez-Guerrero, Jorge, Graham A. Colditz, Elizabeth W. Karlson, David J. Hunter, Frank E. Speizer, and Matthew H. Liang. "Silicone Breast Implants and the Risk of Connective-tissue Diseases and Symptoms." *New England Journal of Medicine* 332 (1995): 1666–70.

Schusterman, Mark A., Stephen S. Kroll, Gregory P. Reece, Michael J. Miller, Nancy Ainslie, Susan Halabi, and Charles M. Balch. "Incidence of Autoimmune Disease in Patients after Breast Reconstruction with Silicone Gel Implants Versus Autogenous Tissue: A Preliminary Report." *Annals of Plastic Surgery* 21 (1993): 1–6.

"The Silicones: Cornerstone of a New Industry," *Fortune* 35 (May 1947): 104–111.

Silverman, Barbara G., S. Lori Brown, Rosalie A. Bright, Ronald G. Kaczmarek, Janet B. Arrowsmith-Lowe, and David A. Kessler. "Reported Complications of Silicone Gel Breast Implants: An Epidemiologic Review." *Archives of Internal Medicine* 124 (1996): 744–56.

Snyderman, Reuven K. "Reconstruction of the Breast After Surgery for Malignancy." In Robert M. Goldwyn, *Plastic and Reconstructive Surgery of the Breast*. Boston: Little Brown & Co., 1976.

Stossel, John. *Give Me a Break*. New York: Harper Collins, 2004.

Stossel, Thomas. "Regulation of Financial Conflicts of Interest in Medical Practice and Medical Research: A Damaging Solution in Search of a Problem." *Perspectives in Biology & Medicine* 50 (July 31, 2006): 54–71.

Swann, John P. "Food and Drug Administration." In George Thomas Kurian, ed., *A Historical Guide to the U. S. Government*. New York: Oxford University Press, 1998.

Swartz, Mimi. "Silicone City: The Rise and Fall of the Implant—Or How Houston Went from an Oil-Based Economy to a Breast-Based Economy." *Texas Monthly Magazine,* August 1995.

Symmers, W. S. C. "Silicone Mastitis in Topless Waitresses." *British Medical Journal* 3 (1968): 19–22.

Taussig, Helen B. "The Thalidomide Syndrome." *Scientific American* 207 (1962): 30–42.

Uretsky, Barry F., James O'Brien, Eugene H. Courtiss, and Martin D. Becker. "Augmentation Mammaplasty Associated with a Severe Systemic Illness." *Annals of Plastic Surgery* 3 (1979): 445–47.

US vs. Forty Barrels and Twenty Kegs of Coca Cola. *Federal Reporter.* 191, 431–440.

Van Nunen, Sheryl A., Paul A. Gatenby, and Antony Basten. "Post-Mammoplasty Connective Tissue Disease." *Arthritis and Rheumatism* 25 (1982): 694–97.

Vasey, Frank, and Josh Feldstein, *The Silicone Breast Implant Controversy: What Women Need to Know.* Berkeley, CA: The Crossing Press: 1993.

Warrick, Earl L. *Forty Years of Firsts: The Recollections of a Dow Corning Pioneer.* New York: McGraw-Hill, 1990.

Weiner, Steven R., and Harold E. Paulus. "Chronic Arthropathy Occurring after Augmentation Mammaplasty." *Plastic Reconstructive Surgery* 77 (1986): 185–87.

Weisman, Michael H., Thomas R. Vecchione, Daniel Albert, Lawrence T. Moore, and Mary Rose Mueller. "Connective-Tissue Disease Following Breast Augmentation: A Preliminary Test of the Human Adjuvant Disease Hypothesis." *Plastic Reconstructive Surgery* 82 (1986): 626–30.

helan, Elizabeth M., and Frederick, J. Stare. *Panic in the Pantry: Facts and Fallacies About the Food You Buy*. Buffalo, NY: Prometheus, 1992.

White, Kimber L., V.M. Sanders, D.W. Barnes, G.M. Shopp, A.E. Munson. "Immunotoxicological Studies in the Mouse; General Approach and Methods," *Drug and Chemical Toxicology* 8 (1985) 299–332.

Wickham, M. G., Ross Rudolph, and Jerrold L. Abraham. "Silicon Identification in Prosthesis-Associated Fibrous Capsules." *Science* 199 (1978): 437–39.

Wiley, Harvey W. *History of a Crime Against the Food Law*. Washington: Harvey W. Wiley, 1929.

Wiley, Harvey W. *Harvey W. Wiley: Autobiography*. Indianapolis: Bobbs-Merrill, 1930.

Wood, Andrew. "Dow Corning Starting a New Chapter." *Chemical Week*, August 11, 2004.

Worthington, Debra L., Merrie Jo Stallard, Joseph M. Price, and Peter J. Goss. Hindsight Bias, *Daubert*, and the Silicone Breast Implant Litigation: Making the Case for Court-appointed Experts in Complex Medical and Scientific Litigation." *Psychology, Public Policy, and Law* 8 (2002): 154–79.

Yalom, Marilyn. *A History of the Breast*. New York: Alfred Knopf, 1997.

Yoshida, K. "Post Mammoplasty Disorder as an Adjuvant Disease of Man." *Shikoku Acta Med* 29 (1973): 318–32.

Young, James Harvey. *Pure Food: Securing the Federal Food and Drugs Act of 1906*. Princeton, NJ: Princeton University Press, 1989.

Young, James Harvey. "Sulfanilamide and Diethylene Glycol." In John Parascandola and James Whorton, *Chemistry and Modern Society: Historical Essays in Honor of Aaron J. Ihde*. Washington: American Chemical Society, 1983.

Young, James Harvey. "Three Southern Food and Drug Cases." *Journal of Southern History* 49 (February 1983) 3–36.

Young, James Harvey. "Two Hoosiers and the Two Food Laws of 1906." *Indiana Magazine of History* 88 (1992): 303–319.

ACKNOWLEDGMENTS

For my dedication, I considered a surgeon, a journalist, and a judge: Dr. Garry Brody was the first plastic surgeon to apply epidemiologic methods to resolve a clinical puzzle. *New York Times* science writer Gina Kolata rejected unproven sources, sought better evidence, and replaced falsehoods with valid reporting. Federal Judge Robert E. Jones appointed his own panel of experts, raised the standard of testimony heard in his courtroom, and transformed breast implant litigation within a matter of weeks. Having to select one of these over the others was impossible for me, but the untimely death of another speaker of truth to power resolved my dilemma.

Silicone on Trial is dedicated to the memory and the institutional legacy of Dr. Elizabeth Whelan, MPH, MS, ScD, founder and longstanding president of the American Council on Science and Health. While she "didn't invent the term *junk science,* she dedicated her life to fighting its destructive effects," according to a tribute appearing soon after her death. Beth and I first met in 1994, shortly after Public Citizen's Sidney Wolfe voiced enthusiasm for a soybean oil–filled breast implant, and I challenged his foolishness in the *Wall Street Journal.* She asked me to serve on her scientific advisory panel for questions relating to silicone, and I have continued my affiliation in various capacities since then. Beth founded ACSH because valid science was too often mute and thus hidden by the shrill voices of phony science, a problem that continues to this day.

Because my work is an elaboration of the writing project I completed for my graduate degree, I offer thanks once again to economic historian Michael A. Bernstein, currently John Christie Barr Professor of History, vice president, and provost at

.lane University, but at that time my UC–San Diego mentor and .esearch adviser. His timely words remain clear: "more than simply recalling events of the past, the historian must also find his interpretive voice."

Everyone who writes history knows the value of libraries and archivists. Although I have worked in nearly all of the University of California libraries, my favorite, not just because it is closest, is the Geisel Library at UC–San Diego. Special thanks to Elliot Kanter who taught me how to search LexisNexis and find *United States v. Forty Barrels and Twenty Kegs of Coca-Cola.*

My protégé and respected colleague, Anne Wallace, professor of surgery at UC–San Diego and director of the Moores Comprehensive Breast Health Center, has provided visual evidence of outcomes following breast implantation given a variety of clinical circumstances.

There are so many others who have assisted me one way or another. At risk of omission, I list those I can recall: Sol Balkin, David Bernick, Tom Biggs, Garry Brody, Jack Bruner, Boyd Burkhardt, Hugh Carey, Buck Cobb, Kelman Cohen, Norman Cole, Ralph Cook, Jim Curtis, Dennis Deapen, Marek Dobke, Trish Drennan, Milton Edgerton, Charles Edwards, Kenneth Feinberg, Sandy Finestone, Jack Fisher (Nashville), Linda Fisher, Joan Fitzgerald, Simon Fredericks, Mark Gorney, Steven Griffith, Jim Hoehn, Peter Barton Hutt, Suzanne Junod, Gina Kolata, Edward Kopf, Carol Lazier, Jeff Lewis, Zan Lofgren, David Luft, Allyn McDowell, Don McGhan, Henry Miller, Rex Peterson, Thomas Pirtle, Sam Popkin, Charles Preuss, Joe Price, George Reading, Tom Rees, Noel Rose, Gilbert Ross, Ross Rudolph, Robert Singer, Melvin Spira, John Stossel, Louis Sullivan, Frank Thorne, Jim Wells, Jan Varner, Thomas Vecchione, Kimber White, Stephen Whelan, and Nathan Zvaifler. Thanks again.

Finally, I remain grateful for the Sager Group and its unbeatable assembly of talent: writing coach and publisher Mike Sager, copyeditor Jean McDonald, designer Siori Kitajima, programmers Ovidiu and Andreea Vlad. They can make the next book seem like a journey well worth taking.

ABOUT THE AUTHOR

Jack Fisher is a physician and professor emeritus of surgery at UC San Diego. After twenty years as head of the division of plastic and reconstructive surgery, he retired and earned a master's degree in U. S. political and economic history. Silicone on Trial is his fourth narrative history, a tribute to America's remarkable medical device industry and reassurance for patients concerned about the safety of silicone polymers.

ABOUT THE PUBLISHER

The Sager Group was founded in 1984 by author and journalist Mike Sager. In 2012 it was chartered as a multimedia artists' and writers' consortium, with the intent of empowering those who make art—an umbrella beneath which makers can pursue, and profit from, their craft directly, without gatekeepers. TSG publishes eBooks and paper books; manages musical acts and produces live shows; ministers to artists and provides modest grants; and produces and distributes documentary, feature and web-based films. By harnessing the means of production, The Sager Group helps artists help themselves. For more information, please see www.TheSagerGroup.Net.